# DECISIONS
*and*
# EVIDENCE
## IN MEDICAL PRACTICE

Applying Evidence-Based Medicine
to Clinical Decision Making

# DECISIONS
## *and*
# EVIDENCE
## IN MEDICAL PRACTICE

## Applying Evidence-Based Medicine to Clinical Decision Making

**Richard Gross,** MD, FACP

Professor of Medicine
Section of General Internal Medicine
Department of Medicine
University of Wisconsin-Madison
Madison, Wisconsin

*with 30 illustrations*

## Mosby

*A Harcourt Health Sciences Company*

St. Louis   London   Philadelphia   Sydney   Toronto

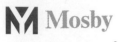

*A Harcourt Health Sciences Company*

*Publisher:* Richard Zorab
*Acquisitions Editor:* Liz Fathman
*Editorial Assistant:* Paige Mosher Wilke
*Project Manager:* Linda McKinley
*Production Editor:* Kristin Hebberd
*Designer:* Julia Ramirez
*Cover Designer:* Julia Ramirez

**Copyright © 2001 by Mosby, Inc.**

**NOTICE**

Pharmacology is an ever-changing field. Standard safety precautions must be followed, but as new research and clinical experience broaden our knowledge, changes in treatment and drug therapy may become necessary or appropriate. Readers are advised to check the most current product information provided by the manufacturer of each drug to be administered to verify the recommended dose, the method and duration of administration, and contraindications. It is the responsibility of the licensed physician, relying on experience and knowledge of the patient, to determine dosages and the best treatment for each individual patient. Neither the publisher nor the editor assumes any liability for any injury and/or damage to persons or property arising from this publication.

Mosby, Inc.
*A Harcourt Health Sciences Company*
11830 Westline Industrial Drive
St. Louis, Missouri 63146

Printed in the United States of America

**Library of Congress Cataloging in Publication Data**

Gross, Richard, 1949-
  Decisions and evidence in medical practice / Richard Gross.
    p. ; cm.
  Includes bibliographical references and index.
  ISBN 0-323-01169-1
    1. Evidence-based medicine. 2. Clinical medicine—Decision making. I. Title.
    [DNLM: 1. Evidence-Based Medicine. 2. Decision Making. —
  3. Decision Support Techniques. WB 102 G878d 2001]
  RA427.9.G76 2001
  616—dc21

                                                                    00-067559

01  02  03  04  05  TG/FFD  9  8  7  6  5  4  3  2  1

This book was conceived as a gentle but thorough guide to evidence-based medicine (EBM) for the new learner. Whether you are a student, postgraduate trainee, or seasoned practitioner, you surely have heard about this discipline often (perhaps more often than you like). You may have finally convinced yourself that maybe there is something to EBM and wish to explore this discipline in a way that is meaningful to your practice.

In addition, your exposure to the topic thus far may have left you feeling that EBM is pretty academic and has little to do with your patients. The perspective of this book is based on the following general statements:

- EBM is essentially about patients.
- Clinical practice is undergoing revolutionary change, with evidence and decision skills assuming a central role for all practitioners.
- The best use of the best evidence yields the best care.

Regardless of your specialty, experience level, or place of practice, this book is intended to introduce you to this new paradigm in medical care. In fact, many practitioners have found EBM to be a "tonic" for their careers; no longer do we look on torrents of information or difficult medical decisions as burdens, but rather as opportunities to apply our new skills again and again.

## ARE YOU A CHAMPION, A BELIEVER, OR AN EMPIRICIST?

I (and it seems an increasing number of my colleagues) have come to realize that physicians seem to divide themselves into the following three types of consumers when it comes to EBM:

1. **Champions**—those who teach the discipline, perform firsthand, in-depth appraisals of research reports, and develop a fairly profound knowledge of the details and mathematics of evidence
2. **Believers**—those who strive to practice according to the best evidence and believe that such an approach is best for their patients, but whose time demands and background do not allow for a rigorous, firsthand appraisal of every clinical question that arises
3. **Empiricists**—those who are content to practice based on background knowledge of uncertain soundness, personal experience, and haphazard sources of new information

This book is aimed to reach those practitioners who wish to become better Believers and those launching the quest to become Champions. The main difference between the two is that most Believers begin their EBM approach by obtaining evidence that has already been deemed valid and has been distilled into standardized, usable numbers by trusted outside sources. Champions, on the other hand, may comprise these "outside sources" and possess the personal abilities to perform the critical appraisal tasks on primary research articles and work in great detail with the numeric parameters to make them user friendly. Empiricists either recognize the shortcomings of their approaches to patient care and use books like this one to become Believers (and even Champions) or continue to practice empirically.

Because any practitioner reading this book does not belong to the latter category, welcome to the world of EBM.

## WHAT THIS BOOK IS ABOUT

The traditional approach to medical evidence ("literature-based medicine") was developed in an era when textbooks (often 3 years obsolete at the time of printing) reigned supreme. The term *evidence* described any fact attached to a "reference" or merely the strong opinion of a respected authority in the field. Although many erroneous practice patterns resulted from this approach, it sometimes worked fairly well—at least for the physicians. With new knowledge raining down in hurricane force, standards of validity becoming increasingly stringent, and patient-informed decisions being ever more the standard, I doubt we can sustain a state-of-the-art profession the old way. EBM can lead you out of this storm, and the greater your experience and background knowledge, the more powerful it becomes.

EBM provides any motivated provider with the tools necessary to **identify** the evidence the patient in question needs, **retrieve** it quickly, **assess** its source for validity and applicability (known as "just-in-time" rather than "just-in-case" learning), and **apply** it to help the patient make a quantitatively sound decision. Of great importance, it stresses the **values and preferences of the patient** more explicitly than have previous paradigms.

I invite you to join me in this introduction to what I believe will be the practice mode of the future. I hope you find that it injects a new energy into your approach to clinical uncertainty and decision making.

Richard Gross, MD

# CONTENTS

# CHAPTER 1

# Introduction and Prep School

## INTRODUCTION

Evidence-based medicine (EBM) is a vital and ubiquitous presence in medical education and increasingly, in clinical practice. As an evolving discipline, EBM has inspired, assisted, confused, and even antagonized some members of the medical community in ways that few of them could have predicted. The premise of this book is that EBM offers some of the most important skills and tools the practitioner can acquire on behalf of the patient in this new era of information.

Among the goals of this book is to remedy an important imbalance in some earlier approaches to EBM. Despite extensive discussion about the identification, acquisition, and appraisal of clinical evidence, the reader often was left with few skills and scant knowledge about how to *apply* the evidence to real-world clinical decisions. Evidence application has been discussed in other resources but rarely with the same rigor and comprehensiveness of the other EBM topics. This book strives to provide the reader not only with a well-rounded discussion of the traditional EBM material but also with strong doses of information on how to use the material in a practical, decision-oriented context, such as in the office or an inpatient setting. By reconnecting EBM with practical, decision-analysis skills, this book strives to target the needs of practicing physicians in community and academic settings. In addition, medical students and residents should find this clinical-oriented approach easier to digest than a purely abstract approach.

### The Evolution of Evidence-Based Decision Making

Rather than emerging *de novo* as a distinct discipline, EBM has evolved from several related disciplines, including epidemiology, research methodology, biostatistics, and more recently, information science ("informatics"). Driven by the continually accelerating availability of new information—from medical research and computer-based access to medical literature—the need for information management skills has assumed some urgency in recent years.

Along the increasing availability of new information, steady progress has been made in the area of medical decision analysis. Focused on the quantitative expression and selection of competing medical options, this previously arcane discipline seems to have found new life as EBM has gained more followers. Decision analysis provides powerful tools that use evidence to help patients, and it allows the patients' subjective values and preferences to be factored into medical decisions.

In my experience, motivated physicians and students can acquire competence and even mastery of EBM skills with proper guidance and sufficient time. However, all too frequently such new skills do not help the patient in any real way, as confused caregivers struggle with the best way to apply the evidence to a clinical scenario.

Evidence may be thought of best as the raw material, or "ammunition," for the clinical decision; by itself, evidence is a vital but insufficient part of the entire process. Even worse, the practitioner runs the risk of assuming that confidence in the evidence implies confidence about the best decision when the two ideas are often quite distinct. To state the situation succinctly, the best decision making in the world can be no more dependable than the quality of the evidence on which it relies, and the best evidence in the world can be no more useful to the patient than the quality of the decision making to which it is applied.

### Example

The presence of chronic atrial fibrillation (a common type of rapid and chaotic heart rhythm) is believed to be associated with an increased risk of stroke.[1,3] Researchers have postulated that this is due to the formation of blood clots within the chambers of the heart caused by relative stagnation of blood in the quivering atrium. Thus a theory that anticoagulation might have a protective effect in this situation seems sensible. However, ingestion of anticoagulants is known to increase the risk for serious hemorrhage (including intracranial hemorrhage, a type of stroke) and requires frequent blood tests, lifestyle adjustments, and considerable expense.

A decision analyst from Mars, where decision skills are superb but evidence knowledge is weak, states that she can build an infallible mathematic model based on the baseline risk of stroke; its improvement rate with anticoagulation; the risks and costs of anticoagulation; the patient's quantitative estimate of the hardship of having a stroke, compared with a hemorrhage, as a result of anticoagulation; and other factors. This model can calculate which decision (whether to take anticoagulants or not) would lead to the most desirable outcomes most consistently and accurately. The problem for the Martian is that the numbers needed to "plug in" to the model are unknown.

The evidence specialist from Jupiter, where almost any research result can be retrieved, analyzed, and expressed in a meaningful, quantitative manner, has a different perspective. He can state with certainty the baseline risk of stroke based on age and other factors and the likelihood of a complication from anticoagulation. He is concerned and aware of the patient's feelings about any of the various possible outcomes or burdens. Unfortunately, the Jupiter consultant cannot integrate this evidence into a coherent piece of advice for the patient because he has no decision-making skills.

Clearly, neither of these extraterrestrial consultants alone is very useful to the patient. Together they might be on to something. Better yet, if either consultant could acquire the basic skills of the other, each would be invaluable as a physician.

This interdependence has not been emphasized in many resources available to students of either discipline—EBM[8] or medical decision analysis[5,10]—although fine works exist in both fields as separate topics. In reality the practitioner must know how to make a sound decision to determine which medical evidence is worth seeking and how to interpret the soundness and appropriateness of the available evidence before embarking on a decision analysis.

## DEFINING THE CORE DISCIPLINES

An understanding of the conventional meanings of the two core disciplines around which this book revolves—EBM and decision analysis—is necessary. Although these two disciplines can be separated formally for descriptive and historical purposes, this book amalgamates them into a single discipline—that of evidence-based decision making (EBDM).

### Traditional Evidence-Based Medicine

Applying the term *traditional* to a discipline with a history covering barely a decade may seem strange. David Sackett, a seminal thinker and practitioner of EBM, explained the discipline as follows:

> *". . . the conscientious, explicit and judicious use of current best evidence in making decisions about the care of individual patients."*[9]

This description sets the tone but may be a bit vague for some students of EBM. An alternative and practical construct of EBM is recalled easily with the acronym "FRAP," which outlines a collection of knowledge, skills, and beliefs including the following:

- **Framing evidence-based questions** The ability to translate practical clinical dilemmas into questions that can be answered through use of accepted quantitative parameters
- **Retrieving relevant evidence** The skills necessary to devise and implement an efficient strategy to obtain the available scientific evidence relevant to the quantitative question at hand

- *Appraising the quality and appropriateness of the evidence* The knowledge and skills required to determine which of the available evidence sources are the most valid and appropriate (the best)
- *Patient-based decision making* The belief that the application of the evidence will result in the highest probability that the patient will experience the most desired realistic outcomes

## Decision Analysis

Traditional decision analysis first attained wide use in the business and financial communities, where investments (such as the purchase of a new factory or piece of equipment) were recognized to produce predictable costs and payoffs. Through quantification of these investments the likelihood of making or losing money as a consequence of one decision path could be judged against competing paths. Analysts did not take long to realize that in addition to costs and revenues, risks also occurred, such as the risk that a machine would break down or that the predicted market would be affected unexpectedly by competitors or technology.

Such investment scenarios became too complex to track mentally, so potential investors developed tools such as decision trees and simulations. Adjustment of one or more variables to solve a "what-if" question allowed for recalculation of the entire scenario. Although rarely perfect at predicting the best path, these decision tools became a formidable weapon for business leaders.

Pauker, Kassirer, and others saw the usefulness of such techniques in medical care.[7,10] The major insights that made them feasible for physicians include the following:

- In addition to the *likelihood* of various outcomes of a health decision, the attachment of a value that reflects how the patient *feels* about each outcome (the value or cost in human terms) is necessary. People associate life experiences with unique feelings and values that cannot be quantified but are critical to their decisions. For example, sudden death may be a very acceptable risk to a patient with a terminal disease who is in severe pain and utterly unacceptable to a young patient with a trivial disease. Because decision analysis is a quantitative discipline, a means to attach numbers to such feelings had to be derived.
- Clinical decision making must content itself with likelihoods, not certainties. Physicians naturally prefer to "make" diagnoses rather than assess their likelihoods. They tend to test to the point of near certainty rather than settling for sufficiency in diagnostic confidence. (How this approach can create problems will be discussed in later sections.)

Thus medical decision analysis is the determination of the decision or sequence of decisions within a clinical scenario that is most likely to result in an outcome or set of outcomes judged most desirable by the patient. (This concept will be refined thoroughly in later chapters.)

Decision trees and related quantitative tools require evidence. For years, such high-quality information was in scarce supply. This is no longer the case, so now is the time for practitioners to exercise their deconditioned decision skills.

## HOW THIS BOOK IS ORGANIZED

The sequence in which the topics of this book are presented reflects my experience in teaching the material. Generally, the more closely the sequence follows a typical clinical presentation, the more readily the reader can incorporate the material into practice.

One conspicuous exception to the aforementioned order is that the chapter on treatment precedes the chapter on diagnosis, a sequence that most readers would agree is contrary to the clinical process of diagnosis followed by treatment. The reasons for this book's order are both didactic and practical—*didactic* in that years of experience have shown that this reversal of the "natural order" makes learning the decision-making aspects of the subject much more efficient and *practical* in that the traditional order of thinking may not be optimal. Diagnosis and treatment should be approached simultaneously because decisions about diagnostic testing can and should be made only after careful attention to the available treatments, not in a vacuum. This sequence has been a well-received, effective technique in previous works.[5]

## EVIDENCE-BASED DECISION MAKING PREP SCHOOL

EBDM uses a vocabulary derived from its component disciplines. Many terms also are used in plain English conversation with meanings reminiscent of—but not identical to—their meanings in the technical sense. These terms are vulnerable to ambiguous interpretations when one reader sees a familiar term and presumes to know its meaning, only to find it used in confusing ways. Thus a brief period of "prep school" is valuable to assure that the reader understands clearly the specific terms used in various chapters of the book.

Terms unique to the content of the chapter in which they are used will be introduced at the beginning of that discussion. The material discussed in the following section is generally applicable to EBDM. It is divided into two sections—quantitative and descriptive.

### Quantitative Terms

**Outcome**  The term *outcome* is popular but not used consistently. In plain usage the term describes "something that happens." It can take on a passive aspect ("watch and see what the outcome is") or an active one ("see what the outcome will be if you increase the IV fluid").

One component of the term's EBDM-based definition is that it describes a phenomenon that is to be *measured* in a quantitative sense. Another is that the word *outcome* generally refers to a very specific end result of a clinical condition, such as death, myocardial infarction, stroke, cure, or duration of nasal congestion. It defines an objective and discrete phenomenon. In EBDM, outcomes refer solely to clinical, "bottom-line" events. In a study about asthma treatment, for example, high serum levels of theophylline as a result of a sustained-release preparation is not considered an outcome in this context; improvement in the spirometry results is closer to the EBDM definition but still not necessarily a "classic" outcome. Fewer emergency room visits for asthma is unequivocally an outcome.

This meaning does not imply that "nonoutcome" studies and topics are not worthy. On the contrary, thoughtful readers can agree that physiologic and other basic research studies are the very core of medical progress. However, generalizing the results of "nonoutcomes" research (such as a specific physiologic event) to clinical medicine presents a challenge. More experienced practitioners may recall stringently avoiding the use of beta (β-) blocker drugs in patients with congestive heart failure because such drugs were thought to weaken the contractility of the heart muscle, only to learn later that β-blockers help reduce mortality in selected patients with this condition. Mortality is an outcome; the physiologic properties of the drug are not outcomes.

This strictness of meaning also underscores the "show-me-the-money" tendencies of EBDM—the focus is on how the patients fare. Thus when EBDM practitioners use the word *outcome,* they refer to a discrete, measurable, clinical event—one that generally affects the patient's survival or quality of life. Outcomes may be trivial or crucial, but they must meet the previously stated criteria.

**Likelihood**   Chances are that most readers' intrinsic understanding of the term *likelihood* is highly accurate. *Likelihood* is an expression of the certainty or uncertainty that an outcome will occur.

Two common descriptors of likelihood exist—probability and odds. The most widely used descriptor in Western culture is probability, typically expressed as a number from 0 to 100, where 100 represents complete certainty that an outcome will occur and 0 complete certainty that an outcome will not occur. All other probability values reflect uncertainty of varying degrees. This definition uses percentages, with which most readers are so comfortable.

Alternatively, the reader may use a 0-to-1 scale, in which decimals rather than integers express the intermediate values. The reason for such a scale is that virtually all calculations and quantitative analyses require the 0-to-1 scale for the math to compute. This text will use only the 0-to-1 scale when probability is discussed in calculations but the more familiar percent form in descriptive contexts.

Unfortunately, drawbacks do exist to the use of only probability to express likelihood in the EBDM context. One such drawback is that probability complicates the mathematics; the use of odds allows otherwise complex algebraic formulas (for example, Bayes' theorem) to be reduced to forms so simple that they often can be solved mentally. (More detailed discussions will appear in later chapters.) Another drawback is that probability may distort the psycho-logic "feel" for likelihood that patients use to make decisions. (This idea will be discussed after a more detailed definition of *odds*.)

**Working with Odds**   *Odds* describes likelihood as a ratio of the chances *for* an event and the chances *against* an event. It takes the universe of possible out-comes, places the "yes" group on one side and the "no" group on the other, and yields a single number. To convert from probability to odds, the following equation should be used; a 0-to-1 scale is used for probability:

$$\text{Odds} = \frac{\text{probability}}{(1 - \text{probability})}$$

Thus a probability of 0.2 is the same as odds of 0.25 [that is, 0.2/(1-0.2)]. A probability of 0.5 is the same as odds of 1.

---

**Examples**

Question: What are the odds of drawing a winning number from a box filled with tickets consecutively labeled from 1 to 20 if any number greater than 14 is a winner?

Answer: Tickets 15, 16, 17, 18, 19, and 20 are winners. Thus six chances exist for a winner, with 14 chances against a winner. The odds are 6:14, or 0.43.

Question: The number on which you bet pays "odds of 11 to 1" and comes up a bit less frequently than once every 12 spins. If you bet $5, how much money would you receive when your number is called? Would you end up ahead financially if you repeated this bet thousands of times?

Answer: 11 to 1 is "Vegas talk" for odds of 11. Thus 11 chances exist that you will lose, compared to 1 chance that you will win, reflecting considera-tion of 12 events. A winner receives 11 chips plus the original chip, for a total of 12 chips. Therefore the 11-chip gain is worth $55. Because you must win once in 12 times just to break even, you would not win over the long term; the gamble pays off a little *less than* once every 12 spins.

The scenario in probability terms might be as follows:

A roulette dealer tells you that the squares in which you placed your chips pay 1100% of the amount bet and end up winning a little less than 8.33% of the time. To calculate your long-term prospects, you might fig-ure that 100 bets (at $5 each) cost you $500. Of these, 8.33% of your bets return $55 in winnings, for a total of $458.15. Your net is $500 minus $458.15, or a loss of $41.85. Therefore this roulette gamble is not a good long-term strategy.

In the previous example, odds are a bit clearer than probability.

**Different "Feel" of Odds Versus Probability** An important reason to consider use of odds rather than probability is somewhat subtle and psychologically meaningful. Odds may depict choices more faithfully than probability in the context of a patient's subjective "feel" for the likelihood being described. The following example may help explain why.

> *Example*

Consider two treatments that cause alopecia (baldness) in 10% and 33% of patients, respectively. In probability terms the results "feel" about three times (300%) different from each other. A patient faced with this decision, however, will escape alopecia 90% or 77% of the time, so in comparison of the two alternatives the absolute difference is only 23%. Either way the reader has a sense of how different the risk between the two treatments can be, ranging from 23% to 300%, depending on whether the perspective is *absolute* or *relative*. These "feelings" guide patients' choices accordingly. Now churn 1000 patients through each treatment and see what develops.

|  | Bald | Hairy | Percent |
|---|---|---|---|
| **Treatment 1:** | 100 | 900 | 10 |
| **Treatment 2:** | 330 | 670 | 33 |

Suppose you then call a meeting of all treated patients, one group at a time. As you gaze at the auditorium filled with the patients who took the first treatment, *one patient is bald for every nine with hair.* In the second treatment group *one patient is bald for every two with hair.* Indeed the second room looks as though an epidemic of baldness has occurred. The "feel" for the difference between the two groups is now much greater, perhaps in the fourfold or fivefold range. That "feel" may be greater still if the patient perceives it "visually" (Figure 1.1).

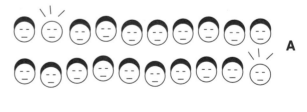

A

**Figure 1.1 A,** For every bald patient, nine patients have hair. **B,** For every bald patient, two patients have hair.

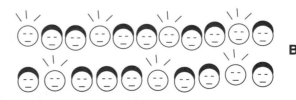

B

Does the difference between the two treatments "feel" more like the difference between 10% and 33% or more like the difference between 1:9 and 1:2? The answer illustrates how the method used can profoundly affect human "value" judgments. For every *increase* in the chances *for baldness* is a corresponding *decrease* in the number of patients *with hair.* Probability fails to consider that reciprocal phenomenon explicitly; the probability simply rises unilaterally as the baseline of 100 remains stable. Odds, on the other hand, explicitly compare both aspects of the changing likelihood. A patient comparing choices must consider the differences as if they were a balance between good and bad; if the bad goes up, the good goes down and vice versa. Odds portray this phenomenon directly. As mentioned previously, neither approach is wrong, but the patient must judge which one generates a subjective feeling more consistent with the choices at hand. Western culture is probability oriented, but an open mind in reference to odds can be beneficial.

**Making Odds Intuitive**　Following are some tips designed to help the reader become as comfortable with odds as with probability:

- Odds of 1 is the same as probability of 0.5 (that is, a toss-up, or a 50-50 likelihood). Therefore odds less than 1 means a less-than-even chance of an event, and odds greater than 1 have a greater-than-even chance of occurring.
- Odds of 19 is comparable to a probability of 0.95. Lots of back-and-forth calculation makes little sense when odds are that high or above. Practically speaking, little difference may exist in a decision between odds of 20 or odds of 100 (probability of 0.95 versus 0.99).
- Similarly, odds of 0.05 compares to a probability of 0.048. In this direction also the numbers become similar when they get that low.

Readers who discipline themselves to work with odds will gain both confidence and a "feel" for what the odds mean in particular scenarios. Table 1.1 provides practice with odds and their relation to probability. The answers appear below the table.

Both odds and probability are quantitatively correct in descriptions of likelihood, provided the reader has a complete understanding of the arithmetic involved. However, a considerable proportion of patients actually may prefer a strictly *verbal* depiction of the risks by the physician.[6] A verbal description in terms of odds may be helpful in communication with such patients.

## Verbal Descriptions Based on Odds and Probability

Following are some verbal descriptions, or "scripts," a physician might use to portray a 15% risk of death. The first is a probability-based script, whereas the rest are odds based.

### Probability-based description
If you take this treatment, a 15% chance exists that you will die from the treatment itself.

## TABLE 1.1
**Odds and Probability Practice Worksheet**

$$\text{Odds} = \frac{\text{probability}}{(1 - \text{probability})}$$

$$\text{Probability} = \frac{\text{odds}}{(1 + \text{odds})}$$

| | Probability | Odds |
|---|---|---|
| | 0.75 | [Answer 1] |
| | [Answer 2] | 1.5 |
| | 0.98 | [Answer 3] |
| | [Answer 4] | 0.5 |
| | [Answer 5] | 30 |
| | 0.02 | [Answer 6] |
| | 0.25 | [Answer 7] |
| | [Answer 8] | 8 |
| | 0.4 | [Answer 9] |
| | 0.8 | [Answer 10] |

Calculate the missing numbers to gain practice with odds and probabilities. Correct answers appear below.
Answers:

| | | |
|---|---|---|
| 1. 3 | 5. 0.97 | 8. 0.89 |
| 2. 0.6 | 6. 0.02 | 9. 0.67 |
| 3. 49 | 7. 0.33 | 10. 4 |
| 4. 0.33 | | |

### Odds-based descriptions
For every 100 patients who take this treatment, 15 will die from the treatment, compared with 85 who will not die.

You are 5.7 times more likely to survive this treatment than you are to die from it.

For every three patients who die, 17 will survive.

Physicians need not decide beforehand which method they prefer as a communication tool; indeed, individual physicians may use both or decide which to use based on the patient. What is important, however, is to know that the odds form, albeit less familiar, is very important for both patient communication and for rapid mental calculations, which will be addressed later. Odds can be especially useful in comparisons of two or more scenarios.

## Confidence Intervals

Various numeric parameters are presented in later chapters, derived from studies of treatments, tests, risk factors, and other clinical phenomena. These chapters discuss how researchers strive, through careful study design, to

## TABLE 1.2
**Results of a Series of Coin Flips in Trials of 10**

| Trial | Heads | Tails | Heads % | 95% CI for Heads % |
|-------|-------|-------|---------|--------------------|
| 1 | 2 | 8 | 20 | 0-45 |
| 2 | 5 | 5 | 50 | 19-81 |
| 3 | 6 | 4 | 60 | 30-90 |
| 4 | 8 | 2 | 80 | 55-100 |
| 5 | 7 | 3 | 70 | 42-98 |

*CI*, Confidence interval.

The overall percentage of heads for all trials combined is 56%. CI refers to whether the observed percentage of heads reflects the true expected likelihood of heads for this trial and is calculated as follows:

$$CI = p \pm 1.96 \times \left( \sqrt{\frac{p \times (1 - p)}{n}} \right)$$

where *p* is the probability of turning up heads and *n* is the number of flips.

make their conclusions as valid as possible. Despite such efforts, probabilistic flukes sometimes can suggest apparent cause-and-effect conclusions when the findings are nothing more than random occurrences.

---

*Example*

A bored researcher decides to carry out a series of 10 coin flips. She repeats this seemingly trivial exercise several times. Table 1.2 presents her findings.

Common sense and statistical knowledge indicate that the researcher stands an even chance (50% probability or odds of 1) of flipping heads or tails for each toss, and thus a likelihood exists that one half of all tosses would be heads and one half tails. However, for any set of tosses the distribution may not be exactly even. For example, in Table 1.2, only one of the five trials had an even split, and some were as lopsided as 8:2.

This discrepancy between the "true" probability and the actual results must be reckoned with in clinical trials. The more flips the researcher performs, the more likely her actual results will approach an even split between heads and tails. Just as flipping a coin an infinite number times is not possible, studies of a treatment or diagnostic test in all patients throughout the world also are not possible. Readers must settle for a representative "slice" of reality.

Does each row reflect the true phenomenon in question or a statistical fluke, such as Table 1.2, row 4? In medical terms, do the results of a trial reflect an actual effect from the treatment or merely a chance occurrence? The key to understanding this phenomenon is the *confidence interval (CI)*.

CIs represent a range of values for a given observation within which confidence exists, within a preselected range, that the results are due to a true effect rather than a probabilistic aberration. Although absolute *certainty* that the findings are "real" is rare, the CI allows practitioners to select and assess just how much uncertainty they are willing to tolerate. In clinical research a 95% CI is used often by convention, but a 90%, 99%, or any other percent also may be used. The factors that affect CIs most heavily are the size of the study population, magnitude of the effect, and "spread" of the results.

For every trial is a null hypothesis that states in effect that the intervention in question has *no* effect on the outcome. (No difference exists between the control and experimental groups.) The difference between the results of the two groups can include a 95% CI, or range; if that range does not include zero (which would indicate that no difference exists between the groups), the findings can be accepted as truly revealing a cause-and-effect association with at least 95% confidence. Of course, up to a 5% chance exists that the result *is* due to chance alone, but this low likelihood traditionally is believed to be small enough to accept.

Conversely, if the 95% CI for the difference between the results *does* include zero, the assumption is that a 5% or greater chance exists that this apparent difference between the two groups is due to chance alone. In such cases, interpretation of the results may be undertaken with some skepticism.

Suppose the coin-flipping researcher from the previous example has a theory that room brightness can affect the outcome of the coin toss. She assumes that with no light the split will be exactly 50% heads and 50% tails, given enough flips. She now varies the room light with each trial and observes the results of five coin-flip trials.

Let us reassess Table 1.2, under the assumption that each trial occurred under a different level of light exposure. Trials two, three, and five have CIs that encompass 50% (the expected result for the null hypothesis). Thus the possibility of "no effect" is included in the interval, and these results should be rejected because too great a chance exists they are statistical flukes; the chance that these results represent a true effect is less than 95%, compared with chance alone.

Rows one and four, however, have CIs that, although quite large, do not quite include the 50% point.* Thus greater than a 95% chance exists that these values are *not* statistical flukes. Researchers and practitioners accept the fact that a 95% chance exists that light did in fact affect the outcomes of these trials, under the assumption that room light was the only variable that changed from trial to trial.

---

*For clarity the CI is calculated for the probability of heads only. A different calculation could be made for the *difference* between 50% (the control group) and the observed probability of heads, but the concept remains the same in either case.

Excitedly, the coin-flipping researcher runs to her boss with the finding that for room brightnesses one and four, coin flipping is affected. Her boss is not impressed. She says that the researcher's numbers are too small and advises her to repeat each trial with 1000 flips. Discretionary tax-supported federal grant money is allocated to the purpose. The results are displayed in Table 1.3.

Several of the following illustrative phenomena can be observed from this more rigorous trial:

- The results for rows one and four are confirmed as unlikely to be due to chance alone. (That is, their CIs do not include the 50% result that would be expected by chance alone.)
- Rows three and five also reveal true effects at greater than 95% confidence.
- All the CIs have "tightened up," or contracted, around the measured value because of the much larger number of trials involved.

Faced with this new information, and convinced of the sound methodology of the coin-flip trials, the researcher concludes with high confidence that room brightness does in fact correlate with the likelihood of tossing heads (assuming no other factors are also at play). If room brightness did not correlate with heads, trials of 1000 coin flips would be highly unlikely to yield the results shown in Table 1.3. Many readers may be surprised at this result (albeit, a hypothetic one) because it seems to contradict what is "known" as true. Readers should consider this hypothetic case practice for keeping an open mind in the face of valid results that contradict current practice.

A final note on CIs and terminology is that when the CI around a result includes the value expected if the null hypothesis were true, statistical significance does not exist. Nonetheless, if the result is a "close call," a *trend* is said to exist. When authors conclude that a trend exists, practitioners should use caution in accepting a cause-and-effect relationship. The use of *trend* usually means that statistical significance was *not* achieved.

## TABLE 1.3
### Results of a Series of Coin Flips in Trials of 1000

| Trial | Heads | Tails | Heads % | 95% CI for Heads % |
|:---:|:---:|:---:|:---:|:---:|
| 1 | 200 | 800 | 20 | 18-23 |
| 2 | 500 | 500 | 50 | 47-53 |
| 3 | 600 | 400 | 60 | 57-63 |
| 4 | 800 | 200 | 80 | 78-83 |
| 5 | 700 | 300 | 70 | 67-73 |

*CI*, Confidence interval.
The overall percentage of heads for each trial is the same as that in Table 1.2, but the CIs are much smaller due to the greater number of flips.

A control group survives a serious disease 91% of the time without treatment. With treatment the experimental group survives 95% of the time, with a 95% CI from 90% to 100%. Because the CI includes the result seen in the control group, it is not statistically significant. On the other hand, the CI just barely includes the control result, so the study's authors report that a trend toward better outcomes is said to exist.

The experienced reader can interpret this information correctly; the "trend" may be interesting but needs confirmation, perhaps with larger cohorts. Unfortunately, a reader less familiar with the terminology may conclude (prematurely or incorrectly) that the treatment does indeed work. A better way to communicate such results might be as follows:

The results are significant at a 90% CI and are not statistically significant at a 95% CI.

This statement imparts to the reader the accurate impression that if he or she is willing to accept a 10% probability that the results are due to chance alone, statistical significance is achieved. However, under a stricter 5% tolerance for chance alone, statistical significance is not achieved.

**Statistical and Clinical Significance**  As noted previously, a CI that excludes the null hypothesis value is considered *statistically significant.** Statistical significance is important but may not always imply *clinical significance.* Clinical significance refers to whether the effect being measured is sufficiently important to the patient to alter management decisions.

A practical approach in the application of CIs is to determine whether the clinical decision would change if the true result were at the low end of the interval versus the upper end. If the course of action would not change between these two extremes, then that result is precise enough for the situation at hand. On the other hand, if the clinician would do one thing based on the lower-limit result and another for the upper-end result, that individual may not be comfortable with the interval. In that case the results may not be clinically significant, despite being statistically significant.

Example

A treatment with moderate side effects reduced the duration of a painful illness by 4 days—from 10 to 6 days. The CI for this 4-day im-

---

*Statistical significance can be defined in many ways. The method described in this chapter is used widely in clinical research. One alternative method is a p value of less than 0.05. Whichever method is used is tied to the arbitrary "strictness" the researcher wants to uphold. The 95% confidence interval and "two standard deviation" rules are used widely by consensus.

provement ranged from 0.5 days to 5 days, often presented in the following way:

4 [CI 0.5 to 5]

You determine that given the side effects, the treatment might be worth trying if the reduction were 5 days (the upper limit of the CI), but if it were only one-half a day you would not choose to use the treatment. Thus although statistically significant, this result is not precise enough for your purposes; you might also say that a half-day reduction is not clinically significant, whereas a 5-day reduction is. You would be (correctly) reticent to use it.

Suppose now that the same study were repeated with many more patients, and the results were identical. This time the result again is 4 days, but with a CI of 3.8 to 4.2 (4 [CI 3.8 to 4.2]). You think that if the reduction in illness were 4.2 days, the treatment would be worth trying; if it were 3.8 days, it also would be worth a trial. Now the results are both statistically and clinically significant at both ends of the CI.

**p Values**  An older parameter still used to describe statistical significance is known as the *p value*. It is related to the CI in that it discusses the likelihood that a result is due to chance alone. It has been defined as "a quantitative estimate of the probability that observed differences in treatment effects . . . could have happened by chance alone."[2] A p value of 0.05 or less is considered significant.

Compared with CIs, p values provide less information for clinicians; they imply that a result is either significant or not, without providing any additional information about the range of values that might be considered acceptable, how "tight" the interval is, or just where within the acceptable interval the measured value lies. In addition, the p value makes clinical significance impossible to assess. The reader is advised to use CIs whenever possible, but p values still are seen frequently in medical research reports.

## Prep School: Descriptive Concepts

**Validity**  The term *validity* is a fine example of how the conversational use of a word can lull people into assuming they understand it in the special context of EBDM. "That's a valid point," and "this is a valid argument for proceeding" both imply "correct" or "substantial" meanings. Although these qualities certainly exist for the concept of validity as it is used in this book, validity has a more focused meaning in the context of EBDM, as follows:

Validity is an expression of how well a study actually measures the effect it is designed to measure.

When a study is said to have deficiencies in its validity (and most do have some), the statement implies nothing about the sincerity or honesty of the researchers. Rather, it refers to methodologic flaws (often subtle) that may bias the results. Consider the following scenario.

Example

A group of patients with depression is identified. Researchers observed that 48% of those patients took an herbal remedy for their depression over the subsequent year. This group was compared with the 52% who did not take the herbal treatment. When a well-accepted depression survey was distributed, the treatment group was found to be less depressed at the end of the year, to a greater extent than would have been expected by chance alone. The researchers concluded that this herbal remedy was effective in the treatment of depression.

The herbal remedy may very well have been effective. However, other factors also may have played roles, as follows:

- The group that chose to self-medicate may have been more motivated, less depressed, wealthier, or more highly functional before taking the remedy. Could these factors have led or enabled them to self-medicate? Were other differences evident between the two groups that could have accounted for the difference at the end?
- A placebo effect may have been present.
- As self-medicators, the group members also may have taken *other* medications more often too, including some with antidepressant action.

Thus the conclusion that the herbal remedy truly is effective remains unclear from the previous study design, as does the idea that such a remedy is not effective. The study's *validity* is unknown; the researchers do not know whether it measures what it purports to measure or whether some other unknown factors may have accounted for the differences between the two study groups. (Readers will learn how to appraise a study's validity with efficiency in later chapters.) The threats to validity are formally termed *bias*. Following is another hypothetic example.

Example

A drug known to reduce prostatic hyperplasia (enlargement of the prostate gland) was hypothesized to reduce the risk of prostate cancer. Two groups were studied, both composed of older men without known cancer who were otherwise similar in terms of risk. One group was given a placebo; the second took the study drug.

A year later, all subjects underwent an examination of the prostate gland by an objective physician and a blood test called a *prostate-specific antigen (PSA) test*. (PSA is known to be elevated in some patients with prostate cancer.) The placebo group had a mean PSA of 4.1 and the study group, 2. Patients in either group with suspicious enlargements on exam results underwent biopsies, as did patients with PSA levels more than 4; cancer was found in 4% of the study group and 6% of the control group. The researchers concluded that the drug was effective in reducing the risk of prostate cancer.

The relatively small difference in the numbers (6% versus 4%) may or may not be due to chance alone. Under the assumption that the numbers do reflect a true clinical difference between the groups, can the results be concluded to actually measure what the researchers state—that the drug helps reduce the risk of prostate cancer? The answer is: probably not; the PSA blood test can be a cancer marker, but it also rises when the size of even a benign prostate gland increases. Because the medication is known to reduce benign prostate overgrowth, the finding that the PSA levels are lower in the treated group, quite independent of their cancer risk, is not unexpected. Thus more control patients likely were biopsied because more had elevated PSA levels, thus revealing more cancers. Had a similar number of treated patients undergone biopsies the same cancer frequency may have been observed.

This study too, for various reasons, might be of questionable *validity.* To a large extent, research study design is aimed at the enhancement of validity. Readers will learn to identify quickly those studies with high validity and seek them out for their trustworthiness.

To summarize, under the assumption that some "truth" exists for every research question asked, validity measures the likeliness that the study actually reflects that reality. Validity is a continuum, so rarely can a person accurately state that a study is "valid" or "not valid." Rather, the practitioner must judge whether a study's validity is sufficiently strong to use for a particular patient.

**Applicability**   A close cousin to validity in the assessment of whether evidence can be used for a certain patient is the concept of *applicability.* Where validity measures how well the conclusions of a study reflect what they are intended to reflect, applicability describes how well the evidence fits the patient at hand. Human variability is essentially infinite. Whereas some variations are inconsequential in the assessment of a possible test, treatment, or prognosis, others can be critical.

| *Example* |
| --- |

A blood test called *d-dimer* was studied for the diagnosis of acute pulmonary embolism (a blood clot lodged in the larger arteries of the lung).[4] The patients were adults with suspicious symptoms who were referred to a consultant at one of four hospitals in Canada within 48 hours of onset. The test was abnormal in 85% of patients later proven to have a pulmonary embolism, and normal in 68% of patients who were shown not to have pulmonary embolism.

An adult patient comes to you with pleuritic chest pain and mild shortness of breath, which occurred 1 week ago while she was out of town attending a meeting. The symptoms improved, but she is concerned about whether she had a pulmonary embolism because she is taking oral contraceptives, a known risk factor for pulmonary embolism. Reluctant to perform expensive or invasive tests, you wonder whether the d-dimer test is a reasonable option.

The applicability issue here requires both EBDM skills and good clinical and scientific judgment. Among other factors, you know from background reading that many tests remain abnormal for only a short period of time. (Background reading will be discussed in more detail at the beginning of Chapter 2.) Because the patient is in your office 1 week after her symptoms began and the study required testing within 48 hours of the onset of symptoms, you judge the results—however valid for the patients in the study—to be inapplicable to your patient. (A useful guideline for applicability is to ask yourself whether the patient would have been accepted into the study had he or she been filtered according to the criteria described by the researchers.) Your clinical judgment and scientific knowledge are critical in determining how much deviation from the study patients you are willing to accept for your own patient.

Note that validity can be high when applicability is low, and vice versa. The two factors are independent. The ability to evaluate both qualities is a necessary skill in the practice of EBDM.

## ASKING EVIDENCE-BASED QUESTIONS

A crucial task in a physician's learning to practice EBDM is to start with a properly constructed clinical question. The exact phrasing of the question varies with the category of information being sought. Specific issues are presented in their respective chapters of this book, but some general principles apply to all good questions.

As a practitioner, you probably have asked yourself many clinical questions, and your patients no doubt have added their share. Before EBM was discussed widely, these questions might have taken the following forms:

Is this a good treatment for this disease?
How accurate is this test?
Does cholesterol cause heart disease?

These legitimate questions address important concerns but in fact can only be answered scientifically if quantitative parameters are found. Furthermore, they lack a critical component of a good question, which is *compared with what?* In EBDM the physician attempts to build into the question the precise type of evidence that might answer the question. This information allows the physician to proceed more efficiently with the search-and-analysis mission.

Although this book has not addressed the details of question phrasing yet, the following amendments to the above questions may provide a sense of how this goal can be accomplished by practitioners of EBDM:

> What is the probability of cure with treatment, compared with placebo or alternative treatments; what are the side effects of such treatment, and how frequent are they?
> What is my pretest estimate of the likelihood of this disease, and what are the sensitivity and specificity values of this test for the disease?
> What is the likelihood of a heart attack in patients with cholesterol measurements of 300, compared with those patients whose cholesterol measurements are less than 200?

The components of questions are addressed in each chapter of this book under the phrase *Master Evidence Questions* in the section pertaining to evidence retrieval. These questions are generic and can be modified to fit different scenarios. The "Master Master" Evidence Question might be as follows:

> In patients like mine, what are the evidence parameters of Intervention A, and how do they compare to those of Intervention B?

In addition to a Master Evidence Question, each category of question has a *Master Decision Question*. In the case of a treatment, for example, this question might relate to whether a treatment is worth pursuing or how one treatment compares with another. For a risk factor, the question might address whether the burden to avoid a risk is warranted by its seriousness. The answer to the Master Evidence Question then is used to solve the Master Decision Question. The "Master Master" Decision Question might be as follows:

> Given the evidence, should my patient take certain steps to optimize the likelihood of a better outcome?

These questions are addressed in the Decision section of each chapter.

This discussion concludes the prep-school education for EBDM. The remaining chapters of this book discuss EBDM as it applies to specific types of evidence.

## REFERENCES

1. Boston Area Anticoagulation Trial for Atrial Fibrillation Investigators: The effect of low-dose warfarin on the risk of stroke in patients with nonrheumatic atrial fibrillation, *N Engl J Med* 323:1505-1511, 1990.
2. Fletcher R, Fletcher S, Wagner E: Clinical epidemiology, Baltimore, 1996, Williams & Wilkins.
3. Gage BF, Cardinalli AB, Albers GW and others: Cost-effectiveness of warfarin and aspirin for prophylaxis of stroke in patients with nonvalvular atrial fibrillation, *JAMA* 274:1839-1845, Dec. 20, 1995.

4. Ginsberg JS and others: Sensitivity and specificity of a rapid whole-blood assay for d-dimer in the diagnosis of pulmonary embolism, *Ann Intern Med* 129(12):1006-1011, Dec. 1998.

5. Gross R: *Making medical decisions,* Philadelphia, 1999, American College of Physicians.

6. Mazur DJ, Hickam DH: Patients' preferences for risk disclosure and role in decision making for invasive medical procedures. *J Gen Intern Med* 12(2):114-117, Feb. 1997.

7. Pauker SC, Kassirer JP: The threshold approach to clinical decision making, *N Engl J Med* 302:1109-1117, 1980.

8. Sackett DL and others: *Evidence-based medicine: how to practice and teach EBM,* ed 2, New York, 2000, Churchill Livingstone.

9. Sackett DL and others: Evidence-based medicine: what it is and what it isn't, *BMJ* 312:71-72, 1996.

10. Sox HC and others: *Medical decision making,* Stoneham, Mass, 1988, Butterworth-Heineman.

# CHAPTER 2

# Sources of Evidence

## INTRODUCTION

Subsequent chapters will discuss evidence—its nature, quality, and use in decision making. This chapter introduces resources from which this evidence is drawn. Several important basic repositories of medical literature are introduced, along with general instructions on how to access them efficiently.

Because we have yet to discuss the details of various types of evidence, the focus of this chapter is general. As specific types of evidence (for example, treatment evidence or diagnostic evidence) are discussed, the techniques specific to the retrieval and assessment of each particular type are introduced. The goal of this chapter is to acquaint readers with the vast treasures of evidence available and help them access this evidence readily.

In this millennium a discussion of medical evidence necessarily must focus on those resources accessible by computer. Readers who hope to benefit from this chapter should acquire (or intend to acquire) certain skills beyond the scope of this discussion—namely, the use of a personal computer to access the Internet with a web browser. Any readers unfamiliar with these skills are strongly advised to learn them; local computer user groups are a good place to start. The concepts in this chapter remain highly relevant and usable, but readers without adequate computer know-how must rely on others to retrieve evidence and may not be able to take full advantage of their growing knowledge of evidence-based decision making (EBDM).

An important caution about this chapter is that its content may evolve. Computer programs and Internet sites are dynamic by nature, and any discussion of their specifics is subject to change. Nonetheless, readers who understand the principles behind the various access methods should be able to adapt readily to the various cosmetic changes that may occur on specific Internet sites or personal computers.

## BACKGROUND AND FOREGROUND KNOWLEDGE

At the 1998 Evidence-Based Clinical Practice Workshop at McMaster University in Hamilton, Ontario, Dr. W. Scott Richardson described an interesting paradigm for the type of medical knowledge that each practitioner might have or need—that of foreground and background knowledge. An understanding of this distinction is useful before any discussion of evidence resources takes place. Such resources generally are not the best places to enhance background knowledge; they are foreground-knowledge repositories first and foremost.

*Background knowledge* refers to the basic, fundamental understanding and knowledge of a topic. It generally correlates well with a person's experience in a given area. For example, a medical student may not know a great deal about the management of diabetes; she must read textbooks, attend lectures, and observe patient care first. With time and exposure, her background knowledge grows. An endocrinologist, on the other hand, may have a great deal of background information about the topic. Background knowledge must be based on valid evidence whenever possible. When this evidence is so widely accepted and of such longevity that it is a fundamental part of one's understanding of a disease or treatment, it earns the title of *background knowledge.*

*Foreground knowledge,* by contrast, refers to specific bits of evidence that are necessary to answer focused questions. The evidence may be so specific or recent as to be outside the realm of background knowledge, or it may be so unique to the clinical scenario that it does not fall clearly into the background-knowledge area. Such evidence often is based on current research and evolves rapidly.

To continue the previous example, suppose a disagreement arose over whether the use of intravenous bicarbonate is appropriate for a patient with diabetic ketoacidosis. Although the background knowledge sources, such as textbooks, might make recommendations, they are likely to be quite "old" by today's information standards, possibly based on opinion rather than evidence, and generally not as reliable a source as is the current literature. The evidence required to answer the bicarbonate question thus may be considered foreground knowledge. In addition, if the endocrinologist has researched this question recently and soundly, the knowledge in fact may be part of his *background* knowledge; the point is that such a distinction is as individual as the scenario and physician at hand.

Figure 2.1, also from Richardson, illustrates this observation. With experience, background knowledge grows rapidly to a point at which it plateaus; the practitioner stays current with fundamental changes but acquires much less new background knowledge. Foreground knowledge changes so rapidly and is so issue specific that the need for it remains consistent. Today's foreground knowledge may become tomorrow's background knowledge.

One of the main reasons to make this distinction is that practitioners new to EBDM who are facing a clinical situation for the first time (including an experienced physician facing a situation new to him or her) generally should spend their initial time building background knowledge rather than foreground knowledge.

To illustrate this point, I am well known in my institution for my enthusiasm concerning EBDM; when a third-year student on my hospital teaching service sees his or her first patient with osteomyelitis, that student sometimes may rush to the computer and do a conspicuous, if inefficient, literature search. Among the first teaching items I often address is that of giving the stu-

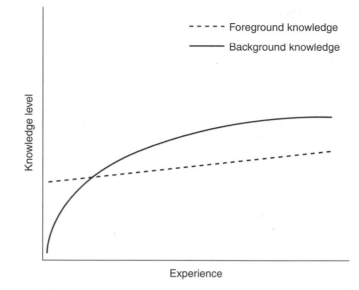

**Figure 2.1**    Experience affects background knowledge more profoundly than it does foreground knowledge. Background knowledge tends to plateau over time, whereas foreground knowledge remains relatively stable (needs renewing to keep pace with rapidly changing evidence).

dents "permission" to read the textbook! A practitioner generally does not "go to the literature" to gain an introduction to a topic.

Another important corollary of the background-foreground paradigm is that it levels the playing field. If a foreground question arises, the inexperienced practitioner (once again, experience relating only to the question at hand) is as well equipped to find, appraise, and apply the evidence as a well-seasoned colleague if each possesses comparable skills in EBDM. Evidence-based medicine (EBM) is a highly democratic world. An authority does not define the evidence; rather, the evidence becomes the authority.

Traditional background information resources, such as Scientific American Medicine[2] and Harrison's Textbook of Internal Medicine[1] have Internet versions available; these online "textbooks" include updates to the original content, thus forming a bridge between background and foreground knowledge sources.

Keeping in mind that textbooks, review articles, and old-fashioned didactic teaching remain important learning tools in the realm of background knowledge, let us turn to foreground knowledge, commonly referred to as *evidence*.

## IMPORTANT EVIDENCE RESOURCES

No single repository of medical evidence can meet every need. Therefore practitioners should be aware of the wide variety of possibilities at their disposal. This section presents several important resources, but other useful resources undoubtedly will continue to become available as readers expand their electronic research skills and new resources become available.

## MEDLINE

MEDLINE is the electronic library of the United States National Library of Medicine. It contains more than 10 million citations and often is considered the definitive source of medical evidence. However, this perception may be overstated. Dickersin and colleagues[3] suggest that from 33% to 49% of all clinical trials were not included in MEDLINE as of 1994, at least in selected specialty areas. Other reviews support the impression that a substantial proportion of relevant trials may not be included in MEDLINE, compared with meticulous manual searching of recognized journals or more specialized electronic resources.[9] This belief emphasizes the importance of all practitioners maintaining an awareness of other resources in their individual specialties and developing competent research skills.

Newer indexing techniques and a growing collection seem to have helped improve the sensitivity of MEDLINE searching (the percentage of all relevant articles that are included in MEDLINE), perhaps at the expense of larger numbers of irrelevant "finds."[8] By indexing in more detail, a wider range of marginally relevant citations will match the search criteria. Clearly the ability to search skillfully and efficiently is an important skill for all future practitioners of evidence-based care.[6]

Once the World Wide Web (WWW) is accessed, a computer user can gain access to MEDLINE in a number of different ways. Although numerous commercial programs exist, this discussion focuses on those that are available widely at no cost.

**PubMed**  The National Library of Medicine itself provides the PubMed website to the lay and medical public. It is available at the uniform resource locator (URL) address, as follows:

http://www.ncbi.nlm.nih.gov/entrez/query.fcgi

Figure 2.2 illustrates the look of the home page as of fall 2000. The page contains a field in which the user can enter search terms. Although the user may enter simply the key words of interest, structuring the search to take advantage of built-in shortcuts and features of the database is desirable. Detailed help documents are available from the various links on the page. A few major points include the following:

- Users may link terms with the special words *AND, OR,* and *NOT* in uppercase letters. This feature restricts the search results to those citations that include either *all* search terms (word1 AND word2 AND word3) or *any* search terms (word1 OR word2 OR word3), or those that exclude one or more terms (word1 AND word2 NOT word3).
- Users may use quotations to unite words into phrases that can be searched as if they were a single word. If the user enters two or more words without

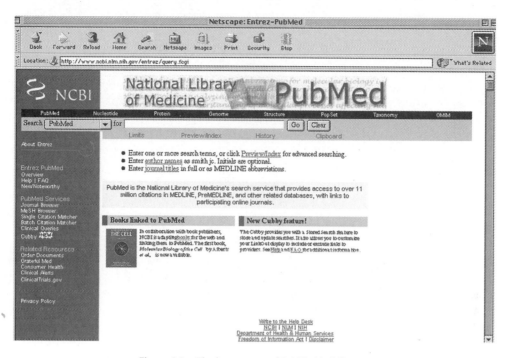

**Figure 2.2** The home page of PubMed in fall 2000.

quotations, PubMed will attempt to match the words against an internal phrase list. If the database cannot find a match, it will assume that an *OR* is the logical connector. For example, a user who entered *Tourette syndrome* without quotes retrieved 1906 citations; with quotes the search turned up the same result because this phrase was in PubMed's phrase list. On the other hand, a search for the term *hospital discharge* found 15,469 citations without quotes and 4146 with quotes; the former search matched articles containing the words *hospital* or *discharge* alone; the phrase *hospital discharge* was not in the MEDLINE phrase list.

- Users may use the asterisk character (\*) as a wild card. This character directs the search to find articles that match the term as spelled up to the point of the asterisk, regardless of the letters that follow. Thus the term *diagnosis* would match articles containing that word only, whereas the search entry *diagnos\** would find articles matching the term *diagnosis,* as well as those containing the words *diagnostic, diagnostician, diagnosable,* and so on.

The addition of a wild card to a search term automatically *suppresses* the phrase-list search described previously, as well as medical subject heading searches, described in the following section. This effect can be to the user's advantage in some situations, but it may create confusing results if the user is relying on the search to find a common phrase only to find that an asterisk in one of the key words prevented the phrase-list matching feature from activating.

**MeSH Indexing**    An important adjunct to MEDLINE searching is that of medical subject headings (MeSH), an extensive list of medical terms organized to ensure that different terms for the same topic are cross-referenced. For example, the term *heart attack* may be referred to as *myocardial infarction* or *coronary*. In addition, *heart attack* may be a subheading of *ischemic heart disease*. If a match is found, the search is expanded or "exploded" transparently to include other terms derived from the MeSH list. This feature is intended to make searches more complete. MeSH helps to ensure that one variation of a given term does not miss relevant citations that use a different term for the same concept. For example, the term *insomnia* is not a MeSH term, but it is associated with the MeSH subject *sleep initiation and maintenance disorders,* which in turn relates to scores of other terms.

Automatic MeSH indexing is a double-edged sword; often the user finds hundreds of articles only vaguely related to the intended search because many have been added from the MeSH "explosion" discussed previously. The result is that the user has so many citations to filter out that the yield is very low. Experience shows that if the user thinks the term is fairly specific and used consistently in medical terminology, preventing MeSH explosion may be wise, at least initially. A simple way to accomplish this goal is to end the term with the wild card character (*) even if wild-card matching is not needed; this action suppresses MeSH explosions. For example, the term *insomnia* matched 5130 citations, whereas *insomnia** matched 3552. Users whose searches match few articles always can go back and invoke MeSH headings by deleting the asterisks.

In contrast, if the user has a concept that can be stated in many different ways and wants to be sure that alternative usages are not missed, MeSH explosion is a good option. If the user is unsure whether the expected term for gluten malabsorption is *sprue, gluten enteropathy,* or *celiac sprue,* a search for *sprue** may turn up 1077 citations, whereas *sprue* alone may find 8069; the former syntax suppressed MeSH explosion and missed the alternative terms.

Depending on the search interface used, a special check box may exist to turn on or off MeSH "subject mapping." Whatever the method, I have found that suppressing MeSH mapping initially is the most efficient strategy; turning it back on if the search results are scanty or if the key terms are somewhat obscure, ambiguous, or unfamiliar is always an option. Many fine literature researchers and authorities would take exception to this advice. My advice is to try both approaches and see which best fits the particular research needs.

**Building on Previous Searches**    Once the user has performed a search, the syntax of that search can be refined based on the results. Reentering the original terms before the addition of qualifiers is unnecessary; a click on the *history* link beneath the search field can recall a previous search; it will list previous searches by number. To add the term *gout* to prior search number 5, for

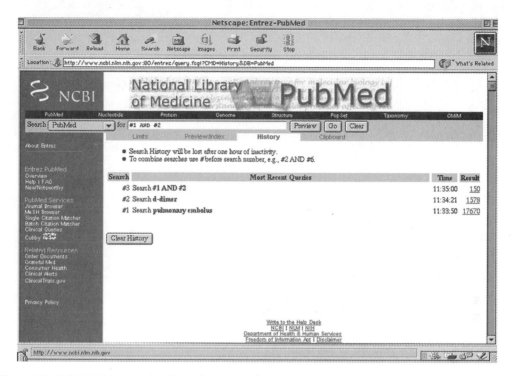

**Figure 2.3**    PubMed's *history* option allows the user to reference previous search queries with a shorthand notation, such as *#1* or *#2.*

example, the user can type simply *#5 AND gout.* The # character followed by the previous search number substitutes the actual content of the previous search.

Figure 2.3 illustrates this common technique. The user first searched for the phrase *pulmonary embolus.* The database retrieved more than 17,000 citations; the next search was for the term *d-dimer.* This search resulted in 1578 citations. By then clicking on the word *history* immediately beneath the search entry field, the user discovered that those two searches were listed as #1 and #2, respectively. The next search entered was simply *#1 AND #2,* which resulted in those citations meeting the criteria for both initial searches. This latter search turned up only 150 citations. Although this example is not a particularly efficient one, it illustrates one way in which users can avoid entering lengthy and redundant search queries. Most contemporary search engines have such capabilities.

**Limiting the Search to Specific Fields**    MEDLINE catalogs articles by specific fields, such as author, journal, abstract, date, and publication type. Not long ago, users had to specify for each search term which field they wished to search, using somewhat arcane abbreviations, such as *.tw (text wording within the body of an article)* and *.pt (publication type,* such as a clinical trial or editorial). Fortunately, newer database technology allows users to search all fields automatically to prevent the risk of missing a term that was used in a field other than the one selected.

In certain instances, users may wish to limit their searches from the outset to prevent turning up an excessive number of irrelevant citations. For example, the user may wish to limit the search to articles in English or those pertaining to adults, or to search specifically for an author's name. (For example, imagine finding all the articles written by Dr. Doctor if you could not limit it to the author field!) Users may narrow their searches by clicking on the *limits* check box and the word *limit* itself. This search displays numerous pop-up menus to restrict the search according to dates, publication type, biologic species, gender, and more. Becoming familiar with this feature can improve searching efficiency.

**Other MEDLINE Search Engines** Services such as Ovid and Grateful Med provide alternative interfaces to access MEDLINE, and quite a few other commercial products exist as well. These services and products differ greatly in appearance, and each offers a unique collection of helpful tools designed to improve searching efficiency. Readers who are fortunate enough to have access to one or more search engines can choose the one with which they are most comfortable.

**Assisted Searching** Many search engines recently have added assisted searching, in which the program attempts to help the user by adding specific search terms or qualifiers to the words or criteria the user enters.

PubMed itself offers such a variation, referred to as *clinical queries,* which is accessible as a link from the main PubMed screen. Based on an important if somewhat dated trial of different search strategies at a time when searching was much more tedious,[5] the program adds highly structured key words to the search. With today's automatic multiple-field searching, search-history tracking, MeSH indexing, and some experience, this type of filtering is well within the reach of motivated physicians without automatic assisted searching. For the less savvy searcher, enhancement seems to be most helpful when the user is trying to reduce the number of citations to those that are most methodologically sound.

Figure 2.4 illustrates the "filters" that assisted searching provides at the PubMed site (http://www.ncbi.nlm.nih.gov:80/entrez/query/static/clinicaltable. html) as of March 2000. The table is based on the 1994 research cited previously,[5] so despite the footnote stating "these terms are as recommended . . . for searches from 1991 to the present," it was compiled before the development of some of today's important search-technology and indexing improvements.

However, users should be cautious about allowing the search engine to perform too many background "helper" functions; experience shows that some users can lose sight readily of the constraints or enhancements that have been

| Table for Clinical Queries using Research Methodology Filters | | | | |
|---|---|---|---|---|
| Category | Optimized for | ELHILL terms? | Sensitivity, Specificity? | PubMed equivalent? |
| Therapy | sensitivity | randomized controlled trial (pt) or drug therapy (sh) or therapeutic use (sh) or all random: (tw) | 99%, 74% | "randomized controlled trial" [PTYP] OR "drug therapy" [SH] OR "therapuetic use" [SH:NOEXP] OR "random*" [WORD] |
| | specificity | all double and all blind: (tw) or all placebo: (tw) | 57%, 97% | (double [WORD] AND blind* [WORD]) OR placebo [WORD] |
| Diagnosis | sensitivity | exp sensitivity a#d specificity or all sensitivity (tw) or diagnosis & (px) or diagnostic use (sh) or all specificity (tw) | 92%, 73% | "sensitivity and specificity" [MESH] OR "sensitivity" [WORD] OR "diagnosis" [SH] OR "diagnostic use" [SH] OR "specificity" [WORD] |
| | specificity | exp sensitivity a#d specificity or all predictive and all value: (tw) | 55%, 98% | "sensitivity and specificity" [MESH] OR ("predictive" [WORD] AND "value*" [WORD]) |
| Etiology | sensitivity | exp cohort studies or exp risk or all odds and all ratio: (tw) or all relative and all risk (tw) or all case and all control: (tw) | 82%, 70% | "cohort studies" [MESH] OR "risk" [MESH] OR ("odds" [WORD] AND "ratio*" [WORD]) OR ("relative" [WORD] AND "risk" [WORD]) OR ("case" [WORD] AND "control*" [WORD]) |
| | specificity | case-control studies or cohort studies | 40%, 98% | "case-control studies" [MH:NOEXP] OR "cohort studies" [MH:NOEXP] |
| Prognosis | sensitivity | incidence or exp mortality or follow-up studies or mortality (sh) or all prognos: (tw) or all predict: (tw) or all course (tw) | 92%, 73% | "incidence" [MESH] OR "mortality" [MESH] OR "follow-up studies" [MESH] OR "mortality" [SH] OR prognos* [WORD] OR predict* [WORD] OR course [WORD] |
| | specificity | prognosis or survival analysis | 49%, 97% | prognosis [MH:NOEXP] OR "survival analysis" [MH:NOEXP] |

1. ELHILL was the search engine for MEDLARS and Grateful MED. These terms are as recommended in Haynes RB et al. for searches from 1991 to the present. The PubMed Clinical Queries Using Research Methodology Filters page uses these parameters for all searches, regardless of time period, in the interest of simplicity.
2. Sensitivity and specificity as reported in Haynes RB et al.
3. Approximate equivalent in the PubMed query language, as used on the Clinical Queries Using Research Methodology Filters page.

**Figure 2.4**   Table of searching filters applied by the *clinical queries* feature of PubMed.

added to the original search strategy without their knowledge. Searches may not reflect the users' intentions as precisely as if they entered the criteria themselves, sometimes resulting in the loss of important evidence. Even more likely in such cases is the retrieval of many citations irrelevant to the intended purpose.

Users who do use the clinical queries feature also should perform a standard search to ensure that they do not miss important evidence. Knowing how to phrase the search query remains the user's best approach. Readers wishing to learn more about MEDLINE searches should consult the articles by Greenhalgh[4] and Haynes.[5]

**MEDLINE on Disk**  The services described in the previous section use the Internet to access the actual MEDLINE computer containing the listing. Users also may subscribe to MEDLINE citations on a compact disk–read-only memory (CD-ROM), a high-capacity disk format that users can access on their home computers. Aside from the fact that users can read these disks without being connected to the Internet, they are generally similar to the Internet search programs in their features, if not their interface. An advantage of some such subscriptions, updated quarterly, is that they include electronic additions of selected textbooks and other learning resources.

## RETRIEVING ORIGINAL ARTICLES

Services exist that send the user a copy of any article (for a fee) that can be retrieved from MEDLINE. Certain institutions and libraries offer the full text of selected articles through their own electronic collections. Otherwise, users may have to consult the local medical library to retrieve the articles. This obstacle to the use of evidence in the course of a physician's practice is difficult to overcome. Services such as the printing of a retrieved article seem to come and go rapidly, so users may want to check with a librarian. Of special note is the National Library of Medicine's "Loansome Doc" service, which can be accessed with a click on the *ordering documents* link from the PubMed site.

In many cases a particular MEDLINE resource might at least include the abstract of the article. From this information, users can make preliminary judgments about whether the article is valid and applicable to the patient in question. (This option is discussed in more detail in later chapters.) In most cases in which the evidence is crucial to an important decision, physicians should not rely on abstracts alone to care for their patients unless they actually have evaluated the entire article. Physicians may use abstracts to reject articles that are clearly inappropriate but not to accept them for patient care; that task requires careful study of the full article. Peer-reviewed compendia of evidence discussed in the following section may provide a partial solution to the problem of physicians obtaining full articles in real-time clinical situations.

## PEER-REVIEWED COMPENDIA OF EVIDENCE

Table 2.1 lists a selection of websites that contain medical information or evidence. Some of these sites are simply convenient lists of primary evidence or recommendations about specific diseases. Others, especially Best Evidence and the Cochrane Library, not only contain evidence but also use very strict filtering standards to ensure that only high-quality research is reported.

In 1991 the American College of Physicians (ACP) began publishing the *ACP Journal Club.* The editors evaluated a selected group of traditional medical journals for articles of interest to their intended audience of internists. They subjected potentially relevant articles to a rigorous and explicitly defined set of criteria as to the articles' methodologic validity; that is, each article was "critically appraised." If accepted, the article then was published as a structured summary with commentary. As guidelines for critical appraisal evolved, they were reflected in *ACP Journal Club's* editorial policy. In time, by virtue of the integrity of the publication and its editorial staff, the publication became a gold standard for relevant, peer-reviewed, clearly presented evidence.

## TABLE 2.1
### Selected Electronic Evidence Sources

| Compendium | Web Address | Comments |
|---|---|---|
| Best Evidence | www.acponline.org/catalog/electronic/best_evidence.htm | CD-ROM, print, WWW versions |
| CancerNet | www.cancernet.nci.nih.gov | Wide range of information and evidence summaries on malignant disease from the U.S. National Cancer Institute |
| Clinical Evidence | www.evidence.org | British Medical Journal and ACP-ASIM collaboration |
| National Guidelines Clearinghouse | www.guidelines.gov | Well-organized list of government-sponsored and other clinical guidelines; not systematically prefiltered |
| CMA Infobase (clinical practice guidelines) | www.cma.ca/cpgs | Canadian Medical Association guideline database |
| Cochrane Library | www.updateusa.com/cochrane/cochraneframe.html | CD-ROM, WWW versions |
| Guide to Clinical Preventive Services | http://cpmcnet.columbia.edu/texts/gcps/ | Columbia University online version of the USPHS Guidelines (second edition) |
| Harrison's | www.harrisonsonline.com | WWW version including evidence summaries |
| Scientific American Medicine | www.samed.com | WWW, CD ROM versions |

*CD-ROM,* Compact disk–read-only memory; *WWW,* World Wide Web; *ACP,* American College of Physicians, *ASIM,* American Society of Internal Medicine; *USPHS,* United States Public Health Service.
NOTE: By their very nature these websites and addresses change rapidly.

Relying on an evidence compendium as a "first resort" carries many advantages. The most obvious is the time saved in the critical-appraisal process. The best such sources usually provide readers with sufficient information to confirm the editors' appraisal and conclusions. Furthermore, the results are presented in a format that helps readers get to the "bottom line" easily. Because the criteria used to appraise the different types of medical evidence are numerous and difficult to remember, high-quality compendia ensure that the appropriate standards are applied systematically.

However, a caveat is in order; the phrase *evidence-based* has been applied somewhat liberally in recent years. Readers should not assume that its inclusion in the name of a journal or article indicates that high standards of evidence have been used. Readers can judge whether such a resource does justice to its name only by learning the principles of EBM themselves. In the end, the practitioner must decide whether to accept or reject a bit of evidence.

Practitioners should make an effort to familiarize themselves with the preappraised evidence sources in their specialties. Before deciding to rely on the research and thinking of a compendium's editors, the practitioner should ensure that the product meets some of the following conditions:

1. The criteria used for selection of the reviewed journals should be stated explicitly, and the journals should be listed.
2. The criteria used in the critical-appraisal process should be explained clearly and meet the standards set forth in this book and similar EBM resources.
3. The compendium should be updated in a timely manner, at least quarterly.
4. In addition to simply stating that a criterion was met, the compendium should state briefly the actual findings to support that statement, when appropriate.
5. The compendium should not be supported financially by any organization with a commercial or fund-raising agenda. In addition to pharmaceutic and medical-device manufacturers, such organizations should include benevolent, disease-oriented societies that could project a bias inadvertently toward research supporting their efforts.

Notwithstanding these cautions, critically appraised compendia of medical evidence represent an important and exciting trend.

**Cochrane Library** Although it is but one of numerous collaborations designed to review medical evidence for specific purposes, the Cochrane Library deserves special mention for its extraordinary quality and scope. Its mission is to review comprehensively the available world literature of randomized controlled trials (RCT) for various treatments covering a wide variety of diseases. Readers can access its complete mission statement at the website http://cochrane.co.uk. This project has even been deemed comparable to the Human Genome Project in its importance to patient care.

Cochrane Centers located in academic institutions around the world accept selected topics to review. The results are presented in a standardized format, and most of them include lengthy bibliographies. Strict standards are maintained for the quality of the research supporting the conclusions. The database has three major divisions—a Cochrane Database of Systematic Reviews (CDSR), which includes the complete text of the overviews generated within the Cochrane Center; a Database of Reviews of Effectiveness (DARE), which reports systematic reviews and meta-analyses; and the Cochrane Clinical Trials Registry (CCTR), which lists many available trials, including unpublished ones.

Cochrane Library is available commercially by direct subscription and through MEDLINE-based institutional search programs. It is a worthwhile resource to physicians whose practices require them to make decisions about treatments regularly. However, *only treatments* are included; physicians who have questions about a diagnostic test or a risk factor, for example, should look elsewhere.

**Best Evidence** A compendium called *Best Evidence* also deserves special mention; it is a resource edited by experts in EBM and includes research in all aspects of patient care—therapy, diagnosis, prognosis, cost-effectiveness, harm, and other categories. Perhaps more than any comparable product available, Best Evidence has defined the standard for how to appraise medical literature.

The editorials published in Best Evidence cover a wide range of topics in EBM and are valuable for all students of the discipline. The articles selected are generally highly clinical in nature and summarized succinctly. When the original article does not present its findings as standardized parameters, the editors calculate these parameters for their readers and present them in a separate table. In addition to the formal appraisal is a brief commentary from an independent reviewer. Further information is available through the ACP in Philadelphia.

## SUMMARY

Advances in information technology and research methodology have made vast amounts of medical evidence available to most practitioners within minutes.[7] MEDLINE is the best-known example of such evidence repositories. Searching such a large database requires skillful techniques—both to find the appropriate evidence and to filter out unsound or irrelevant evidence. A growing number of peer-reviewed evidence compendia are available to make finding and appraising of evidence more efficient for practicing physicians.

A practical approach to searching for medical evidence is to start with trusted, preappraised resources within the specialty of interest, if any exist; if further evidence needs remain, the practitioner should undertake a MEDLINE search. The following chapters will provide more detailed discussions of issues pertaining to specific categories of evidence.

# REFERENCES

1. Braunwald E (ed) and others: *Harrison's Online,* New York, 2000, McGraw-Hill (http://www.harrisonsonline.com).
2. Dale DC (ed) and others: *Scientific American Medicine Online,* Santa Clara, Calif, 2000, Healtheon/WebMD (www.samed.com).
3. Dickersin K and others: Identifying relevant studies for systematic reviews, *BMJ* 309 (6964):1286-1291, Nov. 12, 1994.
4. Greenhalgh T: How to read a paper: the MEDLINE database, *BMJ* 315:180-183, 1997.
5. Haynes RB and others: Developing optimal search strategies for detecting clinically sound studies in MEDLINE, *J Am Inform Assoc* 1(6):447-458, Nov.-Dec. 1994.
6. Heine MH, Tague JM: An investigation of the optimization of search logic for the MEDLINE database, *J Am Soc Inf Sci* 42(4):267-278, May 1991.
7. Hunt DL and others: Users' guides to the medical literature. XXI. Using electronic health information resources in evidence-based practice, *JAMA* 283(14):1875-1879, April 2000.
8. Nwosu CR, Khan KS, Chien PF: A two-term MEDLINE search strategy for identifying randomized trials in obstetrics and gynecology, *Obstet Gynecol* 91(4):618-622, April 1998.
9. Watson RJ: Richardson PH: Identifying randomized controlled trials of cognitive therapy for depression: comparing the efficiency of Embase, MEDLINE and PsycINFO bibliographic databases, *Br J Med Psychol* 72 (Part 4):535-542, Dec. 1999.

# CHAPTER 3

# Treatments

## INTRODUCTION

In some regards treatment is the *coup de grace* of the health-care encounter. Treatment is the final step in patient care, generally preceded by a confident diagnosis. Why, then, does this book present treatment *first* when it usually is the *last* stage of a patient's care?

The reasons are both didactic and logical. Didactic reasons include the fact that the concepts used in the understanding of treatments are critical to the understanding of the remaining subjects discussed in this book and in evidence-based medicine (EBM) in general. The treatment concepts are a bit more complex than the rest of the patient-care process and thus are digested best early in the learning process. Finally, after years of experience teaching this sometimes tricky material, I have found that the learning process flows most smoothly when treatment is considered at the outset.

A number of logical reasons also exist for use of this sequence. The earlier stages in a patient's encounter with a physician, such as diagnosis, do not exist in a vacuum; the practitioner's decisions to perform and interpret a test depend strongly on the attributes of the treatments available for the disease in question. Even an ideal diagnostic test may not be warranted if the available treatments are not useful or appropriate, and a poor test may be warranted when the stakes are high and treatments are understood clearly. By understanding the issues surrounding treatments, practitioners can enlighten their entire view of the diagnosis stage.

Perhaps, then, the comparison of the clinical encounter to a sequence of events is not ideal. A more apt description may be that of closely linked and interdependent bits of information converging on a common target. By addressing treatment first, physicians know where to aim.

Because this is the first of the chapters dealing with any of the various evidence categories, it also is used to discuss a few general principles that apply to all such categories, including the general MEDLINE searching strategies, use of kappa ($\kappa$-) values to describe interobserver variability, and several others. This chapter is divided into three parts, each with several sections to help readers find "rest stops" along the way.

# *Components of Treatment Decisions*

## UNDERSTANDING THE NUMERIC PARAMETERS USED TO DESCRIBE TREATMENTS

In medical decisions, remembering that every treatment is tied inextricably to a specific disease is important. Although some therapeutic measures may be used for two or more diseases, for the patient at hand, such a measure usually is intended to treat only one disease. Indeed a single treatment's benefits may be quite different for one disease compared with another, as might its risks and side effects.

### Examples

Oral antibiotics for nonresistant, community-acquired pneumonia usually decrease the duration of symptoms.[1]

Oral antibiotics for a common cold provide no significant improvement in outcomes.[13]

Local excision of basal cell skin cancer is almost always curative. By contrast, a similar excision of a 4-mm–deep melanoma is rarely curative.

The need to tie each treatment consciously to its disease is clear when benefits are considered, but in certain situations, even the harm or side effects of treatments vary with the disease being treated. (Consider, for instance, that the incidence of skin rash from amoxicillin in patients with mononucleosis can exceed 70%, compared to approximately 5% in other patients.[18])

As we begin to examine the numeric parameters of treatments, readers should keep in mind that these parameters do not belong to the treatment alone; changing the target disease even as the treatment remains the same likely will change the treatment's effectiveness and side effects. Thus the parameters discussed are properties of a treatment-disease diad. For simplicity, we shall refer to them as *treatment parameters,* but this reference always implies the aforementioned duality.

Effective treatments operate by improving the outcomes of a disease. Such an improvement can be considered in two ways—increasing the likelihood of a good outcome or decreasing the likelihood of a bad outcome. Either perspective can be used, depending on semantics and study design. Consider the following example.

### Example

Lowering cholesterol with medication in a defined population reduces the risk of sudden death over 5 years from 1.25% in the untreated group to 1% in the treated group. In this case the evidence is presented as a decrease in an undesirable outcome.

The same study's authors may have chosen to report survival; the "statin" drug improved survival over 5 years from 98.75% to 99%. In this latter example the same evidence is presented as an increase in a desirable outcome.

## Defining the Parameters for Treatments

Some new terms used in this chapter's discussion include the following:

- *Event rate (ER):* The probability that an outcome will occur in a defined population and time span (for example, the probability that a rash will develop during a 30-day observation period)
- *Control event rate (CER):* The ER in the *untreated* population (for example, the probability that the rash will develop during a 30-day observation period in patients not taking amoxicillin)
- *Experimental event rate (EER):* The ER in the *treated* population (for example, the probability that the rash will develop during a 30-day observation period in patients taking amoxicillin)

When treatment effects are described as a *reduction* in the frequency of an *undesired* disease outcome (fewer bad things happening with treatment), the term used is *risk reduction.* When the focus is on an *increase* in the probability of *desirable* outcomes (more good things happening with treatment), the term used is *benefit increase.* Both terms can be expressed in either absolute or relative terms. Absolute terms provide the raw numeric differences between the treated and untreated groups, whereas relative terms describe these differences as a proportional change relative to the baseline. The following discussion first will examine the relative parameters and then the absolute parameters.

**Relative Risk Reduction** Understanding both relative and absolute descriptors of treatment effectiveness is important because practitioners and their patients will be misled easily if they rely solely on the relative. The initial discussion of relative parameters includes several cautions about their interpretation.

The difference between the CER and EER expressed as a proportion of the CER is known as *relative risk reduction (RRR),* probably the most common (if not the most useful) form in which treatment effects are reported. If the CER is very low, even a relatively dramatic relative reduction represents a low absolute number; conversely, a very high CER reduced by even a modest proportion might correspond to a substantial absolute reduction.

---

| Example |
| --- |

Consider the cholesterol example used previously. Concerning sudden death, the risk dropped from 1.25% to 1%. The difference (0.25%) as a fraction of the CER (1.25%) is stated simply as follows:

$$\frac{0.25\%}{1.25\%} = 20\%$$

If the CER were 40%, the same RRR of 20% would correspond to 20% of 40%, or 8%, rather than 0.25%.

Thus a more formal equation for RRR is as follows:

$$RRR = \frac{(CER - EER)}{CER}$$

Both previous scenarios reflect an RRR of 20%. Readers who see that this number is potentially misleading already have an intuitive understanding of the strengths and weaknesses of the "relative risk" concept. This phenomenon also is well known to marketing departments of pharmaceutical companies. Following is the headline text from an advertisement for tamoxifen:[30]

> *"[Brand name] is now the only drug <u>ever</u> proven to **reduce breast cancer by 44%** in women at high risk of developing the disease."*

Although insufficient data are provided in the advertisement to determine which specific subgroups are being analyzed, the cited study[4] demonstrates that the high-risk control group baseline 5-year breast cancer incidence was approximately 1.66%. If the reader accepts the advertisement's assertion, the 5-year absolute risk reduction thus was 44% of 1.66%, or 0.7%, over 5 years (0.14% per year). *Caveat emptor.*

**Relative Risk**　We discussed relative risk *reduction* and *increase* in the previous section; these concepts focus on the *difference* in ERs between two groups. A related term, *relative risk (RR),* describes the *ratio* of the EER and CER for the groups:

$$RR = \frac{EER}{CER}$$

In the cholesterol example the CER was 1.25%; the treated group ER, 1%; and the RR, 1% divided by 1.25%, or 0.8. Note that this number is unitless. RR, like its cousin RRR, fails to describe the absolute changes that occur with treatment. Although more commonly used in studies of risk factors, as opposed to treatments, RR can be used to assess treatments as well.

**Relative Benefit Increase**　Although the previous terms focused on treatments that decrease the likelihood of undesirable outcomes, the discussion noted that treatments can *increase* the likelihood of *desirable* outcomes. When the latter situation applies, the analogous term *benefit increase* sometimes is used. *Relative benefit increase (RBI)* is the analog to RRR; it describes the increase in good outcomes as a proportion of the baseline rate, as illustrated in the following equation:

$$RBI = \frac{EER - CER}{}$$

In the context of the cholesterol example, to describe the results in terms of benefit, the reader must focus on the good outcomes improved by treatment. This goal implies a focus on survival, as opposed to sudden death. In the initial example, survival over 5 years increased from 98.75% (CER) to 99% (EER). This increase of 0.25% then is divided by the CER of 98.75% to provide an RBI of 0.003, or 0.3%.

As stated previously the same study has an RRR of 20%. So, if you were the author, you could choose to report an RBI of 0.3% or an RRR of 20%. Both figures are technically accurate, but they paint very different perspectives of the effectiveness of treatment.

RBI is used when good outcomes increase with treatment, just as RRR is used when bad outcomes diminish with treatment. Readers should be aware (as in the cholesterol example) that the choice can make a tremendous difference on the perceived value of the treatment.

**Absolute Risk Reduction**  When a bad outcome occurs less frequently with treatment than without, the difference in frequency (when expressed as an *absolute* probability) is known as the *absolute risk reduction (ARR)*.

| Example |

A retrospective study in Japan[29] reported that in patients with cirrhosis (advanced liver disease) due to hepatitis C, the incidence of liver cancer was 7.9% in the untreated group and 4.2% in the treated group. The ARR for liver cancer thus was 3.7% (that is, 7.9% minus 4.2%), or mathematically put as follows:

$$ARR = CER - EER$$

Infrequently used but intuitive, the term *absolute risk (AR)* is used when an undesirable outcome increases in frequency (for example, a side effect), as illustrated in the following equation:

$$AR = EER - CER$$

**Absolute Benefit Increase**  You can probably reason that *absolute benefit increase (ABI)* is the counterpart to ARR; it is used when desirable outcomes increase with treatment, as illustrated in the following equation:*

$$ABI = EER - CER$$

The inherent objectivity in the use of absolute parameters, as opposed to relative parameters, should be clear. Absolute parameters leave no room for selective distortion in the perception of how effective a treatment is; an absolute reduction in the incidence of liver cancer of 3.7% leaves little room for confusion. True, this number might mean either a reduction from 7.9% to 4.2% or a reduction from 50% to 46.3%, but the figure is absolute, always on a scale of 100%, and easy to compare with other treatments.

---

*This formula is identical to that of AR, but it is used when desirable (rather than undesirable) outcomes increase with treatment.

**Number Needed to Treat**    An increasingly popular parameter used to express a treatment's efficacy is known as *number needed to treat (NNT)*. It describes how many patients, on average, would have to be treated for one patient to derive the desired benefit and is classified as an *absolute parameter*. NNT is advantageous in that it represents the *absolute* risk or benefit in terms that are conceptually intuitive.

If a treatment improved 10% of patients, then 90% did not improve despite treatment. On average a practitioner would need to treat 10 patients to improve one; thus the NNT is 10. The general formula used to calculate NNT is as follows:

$$NNT = \frac{100}{ARR}$$

With the 0-to-1 scale for probability, the formula would use 1 in place of 100, and ARR also would be calculated on a 0-to-1 scale. By convention, NNT typically is rounded up to the next integer on the presumption that a physician cannot treat a fraction of a patient.

NNT is a mathematic simplification; generally it is not the case that one patient derives full benefit while the remaining nine derive no benefit. Rather, some patients may derive partial benefits, some no benefits, and some great benefits. As with any "average" the NNT represents an admixture of outcomes; it is a mathematic description of the effect of the treatment on a large population. For the individual population, NNT is a probabilistic model of the likelihood of a given outcome.

Some journals provide readers with only the RR and the NNT, in which case readers may wish to "back-calculate" the ARR. Dividing the NNT into 100 to reconstitute the ARR is done as shown in the following equation:

$$ARR = \frac{100}{NNT}$$

**Number Needed to Harm**    NNT has an analog in references to side effects of a treatment rather than improvements—number needed to harm (NNH). The NNH is the dark side of NNT; it is calculated and interpreted in the same way, the only difference being that the outcome is bad rather than good. The equation for NNH is as follows:

$$NNH = \frac{100}{AR}$$

Sometimes, NNH and NNT are referred to, respectively, as *NNH (harm)* and *NNT (benefit)*.

**Reporting of Absolute Versus Relative Risk**    Curiously, the term *relative risk* has been retained as the main treatment descriptor by even such enlightened publications as the *ACP Journal Club* (which, to its credit, also provides certain parameters of AR, such as NNT). Certainly readers already familiar with the CER for a disease would not be confused by this practice, but readers without such knowledge are forced to dig deeper to find the elusive absolute number.

Consider the reduction in cardiac events in normal-risk patients with elevated cholesterol levels. Treatment with lovastatin lowers fatal and nonfatal myocardial infarction rates from 2.9% (the CER) to 1.7% (the EER) over 5.2 years,[3] or roughly 0.23% per year. Following is one way in which a study might report these results:

> Treatment with lovastatin reduced the risk of cardiac events per year by 41% (RRR). The treated group had an RR of cardiac events of 0.57, compared with the untreated group.

This description uses only relative parameters. Another way to report the same results is as follows:

> Treatment with lovastatin reduced the incidence of cardiac events per year by 0.23% (ARR). To prevent one cardiac event per year, 435 patients would need to be treated (NNT).

The second example emphasizes only absolute parameters. Yet another example of an abstract of the same study is as follows:

> The group treated with lovastatin had an annual RR for cardiac events of 0.57. The NNT was 435.

Readers must determine which approach is most informative, but all possible combinations are used. The antidote to this confusion is to understand what the terms mean and interpret them in a way that best fits the clinical situation at hand.

## The Saving Grace of Relative Parameters

Notwithstanding the cautions against reliance solely on relative parameters, an important reason exists to understand them. Imagine a treatment for cancer that reduces death rates from 12% to 9% and another treatment studied in a different population with the same disease that reduces death rates from 6% to 3%. Both treatments have an ARR of 3%, but is one more effective than the other? The first treatment has an RRR of 25%, whereas the second has an RRR of 50%. Without reference to RRR, this discrepancy might not be apparent.

In comparison of results between two populations that differ in their baseline risk or prevalence, the RRR is important. In the previous example when the relative parameters are used, the second treatment's 3% ARR is in the context of a lower risk population; its effect relative to the baseline risk is greater. Readers at least could postulate that if the second treatment were applied to the riskier population in which the first treatment was tested, its RRR of 50% might have generated a greater ARR (12% to 6%) than did the first treatment. In this case, relative parameters *alone* provide insight that absolute parameters *alone* might not. Of course the absolute results would have allowed calculation of the relative parameters in any case under the assumption that the baseline risks were available.

## Summarizing the Parameters

The numerous definitions discussed in this section may be summarized as follows:

- Event rates
  - Control group (CER)
  - Experimental (treated) group (EER)
- Relative terms
  - Relative risk reduction (RRR): (CER − EER) ÷ CER
  - Relative risk (RR): EER ÷ CER
  - Relative benefit increase (RBI): (EER − CER) ÷ CER
- Absolute terms
  - Absolute risk reduction (ARR): CER − EER
  - Absolute risk increase (ARI): EER − CER (for undesirable outcomes)
  - Absolute benefit increase (ABI): EER − CER (for desirable outcomes)

To determine when to use each of these terms, the following guidelines are available:

1. Decide whether the outcome is to be described in *absolute* terms (raw percent changes) or *relative* terms (ratio of two groups) and use the respective term.
2. Decide whether to describe a *benefit* (a desirable outcome) or a *risk* (an undesirable outcome) and use the respective term.
3. Decide whether the outcome *increases* or *decreases* in frequency with treatment and use the respective term.

### Example 1

Carotid endarterectomy in selected patients decreases the risk of stroke over 2.7 years, from 6.2% to 4%.[16]

In the previous example the following are true:

1. The numbers describe an *absolute* change.
2. The outcome is undesirable, so the discussion focuses on *risk*.
3. The outcome is decreased with treatment, so the situation describes a *reduction*.

$$\text{Absolute} + \text{risk} + \text{reduction} = \text{ARR} = 7.5\% - 0.3\% = 7.2\%$$

### Example 2

Combination drug therapy induced remission of rheumatoid arthritis in 36% of patients, compared with 18% of patients on a single drug alone.

In the previous example the following are true:

1. The numbers describe an *absolute* change.
2. Remission is a desirable outcome, so the discussion focuses on *benefit*.
3. The outcome is increased with treatment, so the example describes an *increase*.

Absolute + benefit + increase = ABI = 18%

**Example 3**

Combination drug therapy increased the remission rate of rheumatoid arthritis by 102%, compared with an 18% remission rate with a single drug.

In the previous example the following are true:

1. The numbers describe a *relative* change.
2. Remission is a desirable outcome, so the discussion focuses on *benefit*.
3. The outcome is increased with treatment, so the situation describes an *increase*.

Relative + benefit + increase = RBI = 102% (given)

## Conclusion

The terms discussed previously constitute the final common denominators that contemporary research seeks to define in reference to treatments. By understanding the arithmetic meanings and practical implications of the terms, you are well equipped to interpret and compare treatment evidence when you encounter it in the medical literature. The numeric parameters are the "nuggets" that clinical research strives to mine. The next section discusses how researchers design studies to find these nuggets.

# *Evidence about Treatments*

## UNDERSTANDING CLINICAL STUDIES ABOUT TREATMENTS

Now that we understand the types of evidence needed to accurately describe a treatment's characteristics in relation to a specific disease, let us turn to the ways in which researchers can derive such numbers.

The types of study discussed in this section include randomized controlled trials, cohort studies, and case-control studies (Table 3.1). The significance of observational reports also is addressed.

### Randomized Controlled Trial

The randomized controlled trial (RCT) is considered the most powerful design used to generate treatment evidence. Properly executed, an RCT inherently minimizes factors that can contaminate other types of studies. In addition, it may even minimize the likelihood of contaminating factors that researchers never considered.

The RCT standard is sometimes difficult to attain for a variety of reasons, some of which are unavoidable. It can be expensive and logistically complicated. Even when well done, an RCT is not infallible. Yet it remains the most powerful tool available to get at the truth. RCTs even have generated a robust controversy directed at the EBM "movement." One side complains that EBM goals are impractical and that "EBM devotees pray only at the alter of randomized trials,"[9] whereas the other proclaims that the emphasis on the RCT is no less than an emphasis on the truth.

In my experience, the point is moot; clearly the RCT is the gold standard for studies of therapy, but equally clear is the fact that we likely will not achieve this standard for all clinical evidence about therapy. Evidence based on cohort

### TABLE 3.1
Types of Study Design for Clinical Trials of Treatments

| Study Design | Summary | Comments |
|---|---|---|
| Randomized controlled trial (RCT) | Prospective; comparable groups assembled randomly; intervention introduced in selected groups; followed blindly; analyzed stringently | Most powerful design; control of known and unknown factors |
| Cohort study | Prospective; comparable groups assembled and allocated based on whether groups were already on treatment under study | Inherently less powerful than RCT but possibly still valid; sometimes only practical method available |
| Case-control study | Retrospective; groups with known different outcomes compared to determine whether treatment was more likely in one group versus another | Useful in generation of hypothesis but not as benchmark evidence; may be best evidence available; *caveat emptor* |
| Case series | Retrospective; anecdotal; detailed description of cases reflecting treatment in question | Useful for hypothesis generation only |

and case-control studies (discussed in the following sections) may at times be the best evidence available, and although it bears careful scrutiny, we should not discard it. On the other hand, observational "studies" should not be considered "evidence" for clinical decisions, as is discussed in later sections of this chapter.

**What Is a Randomized Controlled Trial?** Stated simply, an RCT follows two randomly assembled groups of individuals prospectively. These group members are assessed for inclusion or exclusion in the study by researchers from whom the group assignments have been concealed. The groups are comparable at the beginning, but one receives treatment (the experimental group), whereas the other receives an indistinguishable placebo (the control group). Neither group of individuals knows which intervention they are taking. No other differences in management occur during the course of the study. All parameters are measured identically by observers who are "blind" as to which group the individuals have been assigned (as are the group members themselves, in most cases). At the conclusion, outcomes are measured, assignments are revealed, and the two groups are compared.

Let us examine the anatomy of an RCT more closely. (The steps of the RCT appear in italics.)

*First, the study's researchers state a hypothesis.* For example, treatment A reduces the likelihood of a specific bad outcome (such as death) from disease 1. As discussed previously, the premise may be stated differently so that treatment A *increases* the likelihood of a specific *good* outcome (for example, survival) in individuals with disease 1.

Careful statement of the hypothesis **in advance of its testing** is crucial. Although important unanticipated associations and hypotheses may arise during a trial, each such idea should be viewed with serious reservations until it is assessed explicitly in an independent study in which it forms the central hypothesis from the outset. Accidental findings form a rich source of new medical knowledge but should be validated by careful follow-up study once they are identified.

*Next, a group ("cohort") of individuals with the disease in question is identified.* Inclusion and exclusion criteria are established in advance, and certain ineligible individuals are excluded. On entry into the study, each person is assigned randomly to either receive the treatment in question or a placebo ("sham") treatment, which is indistinguishable from the true treatment.

This group-assignment process is highly critical. Typically, each subject receives a number or code on enrollment. Based on the number, an allocation is made to one group totally by chance, as determined by a computer algorithm. These algorithms use specialized random number generators to ensure that the assignment is completely by chance.

For most studies a group of researchers assesses each subject to ascertain whether that person is eligible to participate in the study. For example, previous use of a specific medication, presence of preexisting conditions, or allergy to the experimental drug class all may make a candidate ineligible. This exclusion process is done best before the randomization process; if not, the evaluators ideally should not be able to determine to which group that subject has been allocated at the time eligibility is assessed. This process can be done by sealing of the allocation in an opaque envelope, use of a coding system that encrypts the allocation from the enrollment evaluator, and elimination of any other evidence that would allow the evaluator to surmise a subject's group allocation. The practice of shielding allocation from the enrollment decision maker is called *concealment* of randomization (not to be confused with *blinding* or *randomization* itself, both of which are discussed in the following section).

Why is allocation concealment important? If an evaluator knows to which group a subject has been assigned, that person inadvertently may make a biased decision about whether to include the individual in the study. If such a process occurs in a systematic way, the final group assignments may not be random, even though the original, computer-generated assignments were random.

*Example*

A study is being done to assess the effects of a new drug for the treatment of congestive heart failure. One of the drug's side effects is that it worsens asthma. One exclusion criterion is a history of asthma. Because enrollment of individuals is always an intensive effort, naturally some motivation exists to expedite the process. A candidate is seen who demonstrates very subtle wheezing on exam but absolutely no history of asthma, no symptoms, and no other exclusions.

An enrollment evaluator makes the judgment that although this individual has no history of asthma, a lingering doubt exists because of the presence of wheezing. She looks at the person's allocation to the placebo group and decides that entering the individual in the study is perfectly acceptable. The next candidate with similar findings has been assigned to the treatment group. The evaluator feels a bit uneasy about this individual and excludes the candidate, providing a reason of "possible asthma on physical exam."

Cumulatively, such judgments could result in more "wheezers" in the control group than in the experimental group. Because wheezing may be a clinical marker for a factor that could bias the results of the study (such as mild heart failure), the lack of concealment compromises the study's validity. Had the group allocation been concealed from the evaluator, such biased decision making would have been eliminated. The evaluator could not have allowed "control group wheezers" into the study systematically while excluding "experimental group wheezers" from the study without knowing their group allocation from the start.

Distinguishing randomization from concealment is important in an RCT, but either factor can invalidate a study if not adhered to rigidly; some researchers deem concealment much more important than previously recognized.[20,26-27]

The importance of random assignment (distinct from concealed assignments) is an important strength of RCT design. Given a sufficiently large cohort, randomness assures not only that known factors that can affect the final outcome are dispersed evenly between the two groups but also that previously *unrecognized* factors are spread around evenly.

---

### Example

A study of antibiotic treatment for painful diverticular disease assigned individuals randomly to a treatment group or a placebo group. The study's authors had considered the possible importance of age, gender, coexisting diseases, and diet. Shortly before the study ended, one researcher suddenly realized that a substantial number of participants had had previous abdominal surgery after she noted abdominal scars on routine examinations.

This development raised questions about whether such findings might bias the examiner, confuse the diagnosis, or otherwise affect outcomes. (Internal scars or adhesions from prior surgery sometimes cause abdominal pain similar to that of diverticular disease.) At the conclusion of the study, the data were unblinded. Because randomness was adhered to carefully in the assignment process, the two groups contained comparable numbers of individuals with and without previous abdominal surgery.

This example illustrates a possible confounding factor recognized too late in the course of the study to change its design. Also likely is that numerous potential confounders never are recognized in many studies. Only through strict randomization can researchers be confident that this "mystery" component will not affect the results. Whatever the component may be, the hope is that it affects both groups similarly.

*Next in the RCT process is that relevant baseline parameters are measured similarly for all participants.* Researchers remain unaware of an individual's group assignment and thus of that person's treatment status. Similarly, individuals remain naive as to their own status. This component can be difficult or impossible to achieve for some interventions, but it remains a goal at all times.

In some studies, a "run-in" period is begun in which a placebo or active treatment is administered to all participants, who are observed so that the researchers can determine which individuals stick to the research protocol. The purpose of this step is to exclude individuals who for some reason will not or cannot adhere to the study design.

Run-in periods call for caution in the interpretation of results, especially when a treatment regimen is somewhat burdensome. Run-in periods cause studies to measure the *effectiveness* of treatment on participants who continue to follow the treatment regimen. This measurement may not be the same as the measurement of a treatment's effectiveness for all individuals. On the other hand, sometimes researchers are interested in *efficacy* alone* and do not want to study individuals who would never continue the treatment in real life because of intolerance.

In any event, if a run-in period exists, the researchers should report in detail the number and characteristics of individuals who did not make it to the starting gate (that is, the true study), and the final analysis should provide a reader with enough information to assess how important this factor was. Readers should look for wording such as the following:

> *"12% of patients did not comply with the regimen during the run-in period. Of the patients who completed the study . . ."*

The risk is that individuals who fail the run-in period may have done so for a reason that could affect the outcome of interest.

*After such parameters are measured, the next RCT step involves the determination of appropriate measurements during and at the conclusion of the study.* These measurements are done by "blinded" observers, and the participants themselves remain blind to their treatment status.

**Interobserver Reliability—the Kappa Factor**  Some measurements involve a degree of subjectivity. Radiographic and other image interpretations are examples. In such cases, reporting of a concept known as *interobserver reliability* is especially important. If one radiologist interprets signs of congestive heart failure on chest x-rays more readily than another and if one group's films are interpreted by that radiologist more frequently than those of the other group, a problem might occur even if all involved in the study remain "blind."

By reporting interobserver reliability, researchers can demonstrate that no important differences exist between the radiologists' interpretations; if such variances do exist, the researchers may be able to show that both groups were interpreted by all radiologists in comparable numbers, thereby offsetting any possible discrepancy. The most common measure of interobserver reliability is called the κ-value. Kappa values range from 0 to 1, with 1 implying complete agreement among observers and 0 implying no greater agreement than that expected by chance alone. Values of 0.5 are conventionally the lowest acceptable numbers, with 0.8 and above considered statistically highly acceptable.

That chance alone creates a surprising level of agreement among observers may not be immediately apparent. At the simplest level the reader might recall taking a multiple-choice test, in which answering "B" to all questions

---

*Efficacy* is a measure of whether a treatment works under ideal circumstances. *Effectiveness* measures whether the treatment works under real-world circumstances. If a participant is advised to take a drug and declines or stops treatment because of intolerance, the intention in either case is treatment. Such "dropouts" usually are dealt with in a study's run-in period or through analysis of that individual in the group to which that person was assigned originally, even though that person did not complete the treatment ("intention-to-treat" analysis).

would result in a predictable percentage of correct answers. When several observers interpret the same phenomenon, a comparable "predictable percentage of agreement" can occur. Consider the following example.

### Example

Three radiologists are asked to enter a room and state that a mammogram is either negative or positive. The problem is, they are totally blindfolded at the time. Radiologists A, B, and C thus are returning essentially random responses. The possible combinations of responses are as follows (*N*, negative; *P,* positive):

PPP  NNN  PPN  PNN  NPP  NNP  PNP  NPN

The more often this process is repeated, the closer these results would approach this distribution. The ideal goal is unanimity among the observers so that no interobserver variation exists (PPP or NNN); realistically, the goal at least is consensus, which can be defined any way the study's authors decide, for example, two-thirds agreement.

A look at the possible results outlined previously, shows that 25% of the time (two of eight trials) unanimity is achieved. In fact, 67% agreement or greater (that is, a consensus) was achieved in 100% of trials. The statement that 67% to 100% agreement exists among the observers 100% of the time would be arithmetically correct, even though this statistic relies on nothing more than chance alone!

The point illustrated in the previous example is that for any measurement subject to an element of observer judgment, a baseline level of agreement among observers is due to chance alone, and this level is often quite high. The κ-value describes the level of interobserver agreement *in excess of that expected by chance alone.*

*In the final step in the design of an RCT, at the conclusion of the study, the data are unblinded, and sound statistical techniques are applied.* A comparison is made between or among the groups to determine whether the treatment resulted in differences in their outcomes.

The parameters discussed previously (for example, ARR and NNT) are the ones practitioners should seek from articles on treatment and use in the care of their patients. Readers desiring additional background information pertaining to some of the statistical techniques are referred to the short text by Fletcher and colleagues.[5]

## Cohort Studies

A cohort study, like an RCT, is a prospective methodology. However, rather than following the effects of a researcher-introduced treatment, it follows the course of individuals who are by natural selection taking the treatment, compared with similar individuals who happen not to be taking the treatment. Parameters of relevance are followed over a defined time course, and the outcomes are compared.

Under the best circumstances the two groups, or "cohorts," are virtually identical except for the taking of the treatment being studied. In such cases the results should be very useful, and indeed the method is powerful. Following is an example of how such a study might be assembled.

### Example

Two groups of individuals are assembled in an allergy clinic. As they arrive for enrollment, the researchers determine whether the individuals accepted advice to receive allergy injections regularly over the subsequent 12 months. If so, those individuals are assigned to the treatment cohort, and if not, to the control cohort. When the groups are assembled, the researchers determine whether the groups are comparable in the usual demographic and risk factors, the baseline disease state, and other factors, such as use of medications, tobacco, and other parameters known to affect allergy symptoms. If the groups are comparable, the study proceeds. If not, additional enrollment may occur until the factors "even out."

A concealed method is used to accept or reject individuals for inclusion in the study according to predetermined eligibility criteria. Appropriate baseline measurements are made, and ultimately the two groups are compared. If the treatment group experienced fewer target symptoms, the researchers conclude that the allergy injections are effective.

Cohort studies are often much less expensive and much easier to conduct than RCTs because the study groups can be assembled from preexisting populations rather than recruited individuals. Chart review alone may be the main method for the initial assembly of the two groups, and the participants' involvement is more passive than in an RCT; participants generally just continue doing what they have been doing, the only difference being that they must subject themselves to the regular scrutiny of the researchers. In cases in which the ethical dilemma of withholding of a treatment strongly suspected to be effective is an issue, a control group of individuals who declined the treatment willingly may be assembled and a cohort study performed to confirm the treatment's effectiveness.

Assembling large groups of subjects under a cohort study is possible. This factor lends cohort studies credibility in a statistical sense, under the assumption that the methodology is sound; because of the large populations, cohort studies can demonstrate quite narrow confidence intervals. Cohort studies are used commonly to derive evidence about risk factors and prognosis, which are discussed in later chapters. Their use in treatment studies is frequent as well.

**Weaknesses of Cohort Studies for Treatments**   The most substantial vulnerability of a cohort study is that the two groups may not be similar in all regards other than the treatment under study. Despite the best efforts of researchers, numerous subtle factors may remain that explain why one group chose to take treatment and the other declined. For example, was access to care different? Was one group more highly symptomatic? Are financial concerns operative? Did psychosocial factors make one group more tolerant of symptoms than the other? Are unidentified risk or protective factors more prevalent in the nontreatment group? Not always what the researchers know, but often what they do *not* know, clouds the picture and leaves unanswered questions. Succinctly put, the hidden factors behind why one individual undergoes treatment while another does not can be an important (if unrecognized) difference between the two groups; such a possibility is inherent in cohort studies and may be important in the determination of their validity.

Notwithstanding the previously stated concerns, many powerful cohort studies have been performed. If they are well done, the conclusions of cohort studies may be deemed valid. However, given the choice between a cohort study and an RCT, the latter is a better choice, all other things being equal.

## Example

A hypothetic study's authors aim to determine whether use of a thiazide diuretic reduces the incidence of stroke in individuals with mild hypertension. A large collaborative design examines consecutive patients in several medical clinics. As patients with mild hypertension are identified, some are advised to take treatment with a thiazide, some are advised not to be treated (that is, not to take any treatment), and some decline the advice to take a thiazide, all of which are noted.

Over time, two very large groups thus are assembled—those who take thiazides and those who do not. Meticulous efforts are made to ensure that the two groups are highly comparable regarding other risk factors, such as degree and duration of hypertension, age, use of other medications, lipid status, and virtually every other factor known to affect the risk of stroke.

The groups are assessed after 5 years for the incidence of definite or probable stroke based on rigorous review of death records, medical chart review, interviews, and other methods. Intercurrent addition of unanticipated treatment or new exposure to risk factors is accounted for and assessed statistically. In the end the researchers conclude that the RR of stroke is 0.6 in the group whose members received thiazides, compared with those who did not.

The methodologic rigor and complexity of excellent cohort studies make them imposing to read and impressively detailed. In the clinical case presented, RCTs do in fact confirm the risk reduction from thiazides described in that cohort study.[8] When a cohort study is unsupported by a complementary RCT, the cohort study may provide the best evidence available and can serve as benchmark evidence if it is valid and applicable. However, an RCT is always desirable to confirm the evidence provided by a cohort study.

**Case-Control Studies** Case-control studies are used rarely for treatment trials nowadays. They are more common in studies of risk factors, and a detailed discussion of their methodology is presented in Chapter 5. Such studies are mentioned in this chapter only because practitioners may encounter case-control studies occasionally in the search for treatment evidence.

**Case Series and Case Reports** Students of medical history may marvel at the exquisite case reports that mark the clinical publications of Osler and others. At the stage in which disease categorization and prognosis were the mainstays of medical science, such works contributed greatly to the common knowledge. Powers of observation were admired and cultivated in medical circles.

Even today, the very first reports of new diseases often are marked by such case series. Toxic shock syndrome and acquired immunodeficiency syndrome are examples of recently described entities in which such reports surfaced. From these careful reports often emerge patterns that prompt speculation and hypotheses, which then can be tested.

| *Example* |

The abstract and conclusion of an article on the use of abdominal ultrasound after abdominoplasty (fat removal with liposuction) state the following:

*"This method, if performed routinely postabdominoplasty, will aid the surgeon in managing potential complications such as wound-healing problems, infection, and patient discomfort. . . . We recommend the routine utilization of ultrasound in patients undergoing abdominoplasty."*[19]

This self-described 6-year prospective study outlines 80 procedures with their complication rates. It notes that ultrasound was obtained in 70% of patients and often identified fluid and blood collections.

Final outcomes between the group that underwent ultrasound and the group that did not are not compared. Their baseline characteristics and risks for complications are not addressed. This diagnostic test is treated as though it were a treatment in the context of the article's conclusions. The researcher apparently was fully aware of the results of the ultrasound (that is, not blind to the patients' test status). No quantitative data are presented to describe its benefits. For this and many other reasons, the validity of the study's potentially costly conclusions apparently is not supported by its findings or its methodology.

An important point to stress is that *case reports should not be viewed as medical evidence.* As tools for confirming the effectiveness of treatment or other evidence, they claim no validity. Practitioners should not assume such reports are valid even when they represent the only literature available. The sometimes pseudoscientific language and occasionally presumptuous conclusions of case reports may lend their readers the impression of authority but add little to medical evidence. A case series is viewed best as the sharing of observations.

## Summary

This section described the methodology for the study of treatments. The RCT, with all its complexity and rigor, is the best method for the study of treatments. Cohort studies also are powerful tools, although less so. However, practitioners must observe caution in relying on observational and case-control studies.

# RETRIEVING EVIDENCE ABOUT TREATMENTS

## The Master Evidence Question

The Master Evidence Question for treatment is as follows:

*What are the frequencies of the side effects and disease outcome improvements in treated patients, compared with those who did not receive treatment?*

The evidence may take the form of AR, RR, or NNT. Knowing the types of study design used in treatment outcomes research, the reader can understand why the strategies best used to find treatment evidence are those designed to retrieve RCTs whenever possible. Other types of research also may be desirable in case the former are not available. Because the vast medical literature contains seemingly unlimited numbers of reports that are of less use or lower quality than the RCT, the reader's search strategy must filter out such reports to prevent having to sift through hundreds or thousands of poor-quality articles.

Readers may want to refer to the section in Chapter 2 on the basics of searching for evidence and information on evidence resources and the skills needed to use them. Although the following discussion refers to MEDLINE searching, readers first should search those databases of preappraised evidence relevant to the specialty area at hand. For example, in the case of therapy questions, an initial search of Cochrane and Best Evidence is advised. Only if the results are inadequate would the search progress to MEDLINE.

Now let us see how to search MEDLINE when the need arises. (Readers should remember to *search Cochrane and Best Evidence first*. In addition, particular specialties may have equivalent resources that may provide excellent initial searches.)

> NOTE: The search strategies discussed in this and other chapters are adaptations of the research done by Haynes[10] in 1994. At that time, search engines often required the user to specify the field being searched; indexing was less consistent, and sequential searching was more cumbersome. The results of the study were of great interest, but the strategies were complex and unwieldy. The approach presented in the following discussion strives to take advantage of the insights in that original research by use of simpler strategies available with current database technology and indexing. Considerable trial-and-error and experiential components are unavoidable in effective searching, so the reader is

advised to practice searching at every opportunity and develop a systematic approach. Readers may find a review of the general searching discussion in Chapter 2 useful.

## The Two-Pass Search Strategy

This section's initial discussion focuses on the "two-pass" search strategy, which is repeated in subsequent chapters concerning types other than treatment evidence. The underlying concept is to use the first "pass," or search, to retrieve as many reasonably relevant articles as possible, with the understanding that many such articles may not be high quality or appropriate. Because the user does not know how successful the first pass will be, the search should err on the side of producing results that may be too broad. In literature searching, the ability of a search to retrieve the highest percentage of available citations on a topic is considered its *sensitivity.*

The second pass is used to refine the results of the first pass. Its purpose is to narrow the field to include those citations most likely to concern RCTs. If the number of citations from the first pass is small, the second pass may be unnecessary. If it is large, the second pass often is helpful.

Although the specific syntax of each pass will be described, an initial examination of the possible reasons why the first pass may not retrieve as many articles as the user may need is in order. The most obvious reason is that many research reports simply do not exist on that topic. Another reason may be that the search term used is too narrow or even incorrect (not infrequently because of typographic error). Users who encounter such a "dry tap" on the first pass (assuming the entry was typed correctly) may choose to enable subject matching by using the MeSH index (medical subject heading) described in Chapter 2. Perhaps the indexers used a different term for the topic at hand; the MeSH index will probably cross-reference the user's term to its subject heading.

A final caution is to use parentheses carefully; a search for *x AND (y OR z)* is quite different from *x AND y OR z*. The first example is interpreted to encompass articles containing x and *from those,* the finding of articles containing either y or z, whereas the second example instructs the database to find articles containing both x and y and then start from scratch to find articles containing z and add them to the first batch.

If these steps still fail to yield a meaningful number of articles, the user may apply clinical knowledge to rephrase the index term or consult with more experienced colleagues. Effective searching is a knack that grows with experience.

## Two-Pass Syntax for Treatment Evidence

For pass 1 the user types the root-word fragments *random* and *therap*. With wild-card syntax the terms become *random** and *therap** (asterisks or whichever wild-card character the search engine uses, such as $ or # ). This use encompasses the terms *randomized, random, randomization, therapy,* and *therapeutic.* The search engine should be set to search *all* fields, including abstract, text, title, and so on.

This strategy should find almost all articles of interest in most cases, under the assumption that randomization is considered a criterion. For example, to search for studies about the drug nifedipine used to treat hypertension (remembering that all treatment studies are actually treatment-disease diad studies), the user might try the following syntax:

nifedipine AND hypertension AND (random* OR therap*)

This query in the PubMed database yielded 1536 citations.

Parentheses are included for the last two terms to ensure that the search engine does not interpret the latter terms to mean that it should find articles containing the words *nifedipine* and *hypertension* and *random** and add to them all articles that include the term *therap**. With parentheses the search unambiguously instructs the database to find articles containing both *nifedipine* and *hypertension* and from those, select the ones also containing either the term *random** or *therap**.

Few physicians could spare the time to search all 1536 articles. The next goal is to narrow the number of citations to those most likely to yield high-quality evidence. Thus the following discussion focuses on the second pass. The syntax is designed to qualify the search to include the full phrase *randomized controlled trial*. The exact query is as follows:

#1 AND "randomized controlled trial"

Use of the following special notations should be observed:

- **#1**—PubMed understands that when a query has been completed, its results may be referred to with the pound sign (#), followed by a number assigned to that query. (A click on the *history* link in the PubMed window allows the user to see a list of previous queries and their respective numbers.) This feature provides a shortcut to avoid reentry of the full syntax of pass 1.
- **Quotation marks**—This notation ties the included words together into one concept that is treated as a single word. Without the quotes, some search engines might treat the three words as separate search criteria (randomized OR controlled OR trial). Because of its phrase lists and other protocols, PubMed does not "care" whether this example contains quotes, but the use of quotation marks is a good habit to ensure that the search proceeds as the user intends in any search engine.

In the most previous example, pass 2 narrowed the list of citations to 463 articles, a number much more practical than 1536; however, 436 is still an impractical number of articles for a physician to consult while the patient waits in the exam room. The following tips apply when even pass 2 yields more articles than the user can handle conscientiously:

- A search for citations in which the key word is included in the *title* of the article is useful, in which case the entry would appear as follows:

#2 AND nifedipine

- Before searching, the user should activate the *limits* link to limit the search to the title word.

  *Results:* 322 citations

If pass 2 had yielded too small a number of citations, the search may focus on an area in which few RCTs exist; a tip to increase the number of results is to add the phrase *OR cohort* to the query to find relevant cohort studies.

If despite the user's best efforts the result still yields too many citations to sort through, a few options exist. Generally the articles are listed in reverse chronologic order. Thus of the 322 citations, the 40th citation is already almost 3 years old. The user can judge how far back the results remain relevant. Another approach is to limit the search to only those citations with abstracts; although this option does not filter quality, it does make the task more efficient as long as the user is aware that some evidence lacking an abstract in the citation may be overlooked.

A review of the 322 citations reveals quite a few dealing with pregnancy and emergencies; by searching with the phrase *#5 NOT pregnancy NOT emergenc\** the user can narrow the results further to 293 citations. Similar exclusions may be used to reduce the list appropriately.

At some point the law of diminishing returns will lead the user to stop searching and start reviewing the narrowed list of citations. The treatment search strategy may be summarized as follows:

**Pass 1:** Keywords AND (random\* or therap\*)
  *Just right:* Search may be complete.
  *Too few:* Check for errors; try different words; activate MeSH referencing by eliminating all wild cards.
  *Too many:* Proceed to pass 2.
**Pass 2:** Results of pass 1 AND "randomized controlled trial"
  *Just right:* Search is complete.
  *Too few:* Try pass 2 but add *OR cohort.*
  *Too many:* Search for key words in title field; use *limit* options; scan citations to exclude the obvious incidental retrievals using *NOT.* Scan citations back in time as far as you feel the topic warrants.

## JUDGING THE SUITABILITY OF TREATMENT EVIDENCE

The term *suitability* in this discussion describes the appropriateness of the use of the results of a study in the care of an individual patient. For a study to be suitable for a patient it must meet at least two general criteria—validity and applicability, both of which are defined in Chapter 1. If a study is not valid, it is not suitable for any patient. If a study is valid, the practitioner must determine whether it is applicable to a given patient. Furthermore, if the study is applicable, it may be suitable for that patient but not necessarily for a different patient.

Even if the practitioner deems a treatment suitable for a certain patient, that practitioner may not necessarily want to proceed with it. The missing ingredient is whether the risks and benefits of the "suitable" treatment are favorable to the patient. (This separate and critical component of the decision is addressed in the later section on decision making.)

Until several years ago the way research was reported in journals was inconsistent, and gleaning of the necessary elements to determine suitability required a focused, detailed reading of the article (sometimes several times). Fortunately, two trends have made the task much more efficient in recent years—inclusion of the requisite evidence within the abstract itself and growth of peer-reviewed compendia of the literature, in which trained reviewers have performed much of the assessment on behalf of the physician (at least in terms of validity). However, developing the skills necessary to assess suitability remains important for each practitioner because many important research reports exist that do not contain the requisite evidence and have not been reviewed by professionals.

Traditional teaching of EBM[24-25] refers to the process by which suitability is determined as "critical appraisal." This step generally consists of the initial assessment of validity followed by that of applicability. Although the sequence means little to the practitioner who plans to appraise both components, for maximal efficiency in a busy clinical scenario the appraisal of applicability before validity is best. The reason for this reversal is that assessment of applicability is generally faster and more straightforward; if applicability is poor, the suitability of the evidence can be dismissed immediately without assessment of the validity. However, if the practitioner has both the time and the ability, both components should be assessed.

The assessment sequence is shown graphically in Figure 3.1. This illustration serves as a map for the subsequent discussion, in which the specific terms and rules of assessment are described.

## Applicability

Applicability, as noted, assesses how well the results of a study apply to a particular patient; conversely, the practitioner may ask how well the patient fits the study group.

### Does the Study Fit My Patient from Biographic and Biologic Perspectives?

The practitioner's clinical judgment and experience are crucial in determining just how much deviation in either category is acceptable. In this context, *biographic* refers to the patient's age, gender, and perhaps social-risk profile. *Biologic* refers to biologic risk profile, disease type and stage, and similar clinical factors that can affect the treatment outcome. Examples of each type can clarify the procedure.

| Example 1 |

A study of the use of tacrine to treat individuals with Alzheimer's disease demonstrated that 27% improved with treatment, compared with 17% in the control group.[14] Up to 43% of participants dropped out of the

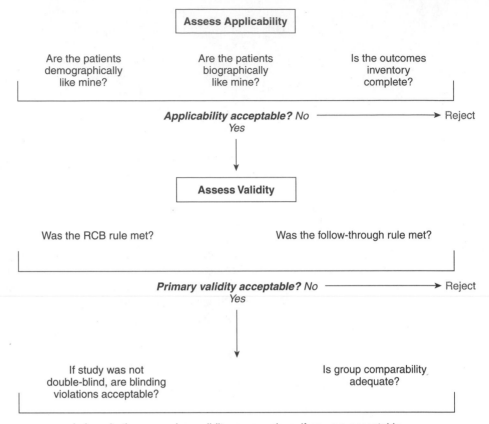

**Figure 3.1**    Map of steps used to perform a critical appraisal of evidence regarding treatment. Note that *accept* and *reject* are rarely absolute but rather reflect the extremes of how closely a finding is likely to approximate the "true" effect. *RCB,* Random, concealed, blind.

study because of drug intolerance. The subjects had a mean age of 73 years, 53% of whom were women with mild to moderate disease. Exclusions included significant cardiac disease, stroke, diabetes, liver, or kidney disease.

Your patient is a 62-year-old man with diabetes who has experienced several transient ischemic episodes in the past year. Epidemiologically, you determine that he is younger than the study group; you judge this deviation to be important but assume that it is not a "show-stopper" (that is, a disqualifier) because Alzheimer's disease is not known to be biologically different in younger individuals, compared with older ones. The presence of diabetes also is important because the study did not include any individuals with the disease. Again, this deviation is a concern, but given the limited treatment options and high stakes of the treatment decision, you might be willing to tolerate it.

Finally, you note that ischemic cerebral disease was excluded. Your patient clearly has this condition; it is an important cause of dementia that might manifest itself much like Alzheimer's disease and in fact is a strong possibility as a cause or contributor to your patient's dementia. You deem this last factor to be biologically important enough to judge the results inapplicable to your patient. Weighing the other concerns and poor tolerance of the drug among participants, you conclude that the study's evidence was insufficient to warrant recommending the drug for your patient.

### Example 2

A study of two strategies for blood transfusion in the intensive care setting looked at 838 individuals (mean age of 58 years, 63% of them men) with initial hemoglobin levels less than 9 g/dl.[12] Exclusions included current active hemorrhage, brain death or imminent death, and routine admission after coronary bypass surgery. One group received blood sufficient to maintain the hemoglobin in the 7-to-9 g/dl range. The other group maintained a range from 10 to 12 g/dl. All-cause mortality at 30 days, length of stay in the hospital and in intensive care, 60 day mortality, and organ system failure rates were similar. The "7-to-9 range" group had 7% fewer episodes of cardiac events and 6% fewer episodes of pulmonary edema.

Your patient is a 54-year-old woman who went to the emergency room having vomited blood 2 hours previous and complained of black, tarry stools the day before. She had a myocardial infarction 3 years ago and smokes two packs of cigarettes daily. Her hemoglobin level on admission to the intensive care unit is 6 g/dl. Her stools are melanotic, and nasogastric aspirate shows coffee ground-like matter. You determine the target hemoglobin level as you initiate transfusions.

On appraising the study for applicability, you note that the patient is in the correct age group (that is, that represented in the study) and that women were represented adequately in the study. The clinical criteria are partially met by the patient's symptoms, but you judge that your patient may be bleeding *actively* based on the clinical findings. Her known coronary disease is also a concern, and you analyze the study to see whether individuals with coronary disease were studied separately, concluding that insufficient data exists. Although the demographic applicability seems acceptable, you reason that unlike the participants in the study, your patient is bleeding actively and thus may require a higher hemoglobin "reserve" on which to depend. You also have reservations about her coronary disease rendering her vulnerable to anemia-related myocardial ischemia. Although the risk of heart failure rises with the more aggressive transfusion strategy, you judge this risk to be clinically acceptable. Thus you judge the study to be inapplicable to this patient and aim for a hemoglobin level in the 10-to-12 g/dl range.

| *Example 3* |

A study examined the effect of biennial fecal occult blood screening on colon cancer mortality over almost 8 years.[11] More than 44,000 adults of both sexes ages 45 to 74 years received screening and were compared with a group of approximately 76,000 who did not receive screening. The screened group of individuals with colon cancer had an 18% reduction in mortality. This 18% reduction in individuals with colon cancer yielded an overall reduction for all those screened of less than 0.5% because only a small fraction of screened subjects developed cancer.

Your patient is a 40-year-old man receiving periodic screening evaluations. You wonder whether the results of the aforementioned colon-cancer study would support biennial fecal occult blood testing for him. Although this complex study has numerous validity issues requiring careful scrutiny, you focus on applicability. Noting the age range of 45 to 74 years and knowing that the incidence of colon cancer increases with age, you hesitate. Further noting that the overall effect on mortality for the entire screened group (as opposed to the group that ultimately developed cancer) was small, you presume that your patient would derive very little benefit from such screening at age 40. Finally, you know that a high percentage of positive tests in this setting do not represent precancerous adenomata, and you appreciate the importance of cost and anxiety associated with unnecessary colonoscopy for false-positive results.

Without even assessing its validity, you decide not to accept this study to support biennial fecal occult blood screening for your patient; its applicability is too low.

### Is the Outcome Inventory Sufficiently Complete for My Patient?

If a study is highly applicable to your patient from biologic and biographic perspectives, the inclusion in the study of all the important outcomes of a treatment and its target disease is important. For example, a study of prostate surgery in elderly men may be highly applicable to your patient in terms of symptom relief, incontinence, and patient demographics; however, the same study may fail to report the incidence of impotence. If your patient considers this condition important, you may not be able to use that otherwise highly applicable study. On the other hand, use of the study's results may be suitable on a comparable patient for whom impotence is a far less important issue. The outcome inventory should be assessed not only for side effects but also for symptoms that are improved.

## Validity

As discussed in Chapter 1, *validity* refers to how well a research study measures the phenomena it strives to measure. The two categories of validity criteria (primary and secondary) define whether the conditions to be met are mandatory for the study to be considered acceptable (primary) or important but not necessarily required (secondary).

**Primary Validity Criteria**  The criteria discussed in the following section may be considered necessary for the acceptance of a study as valid. If these criteria are not met, the evidence generally should not be relied on for patient decision making.

*The RCB rule*  Were the subjects enrolled and assigned to their respective groups in a manner that was *R*andom, *C*oncealed, and *B*lind? (The meanings of these criteria are discussed in Chapter 1.)

Each practitioner must determine from the article whether the group assignment process was truly *random,* such as by a computer-generated random number scheme; whether this random allocation was *concealed* from those researchers responsible for assessing individuals for enrollment; and whether the researchers were *blind* as to which group the individuals were assigned during the study. As discussed in the following section, blinding is a relative criterion, and its absence may be acceptable in some situations.

The practitioner who is confident that one or more of these three requirements is lacking cannot rely on the validity of the study. This guideline does not mean that the results or conclusions of the study are necessarily incorrect, nor that certain subsets of information within the study may not be valid; however, it does mean that the methodology or its implementation is vulnerable to systematic distortion and contamination of the results to a degree that those results may not reflect the "truth."

| Example | *Randomization* |
|---|---|

A study of the effect of a new sleeping pill involves the enrollment of adults who visited an evening clinic. Preprinted packets are distributed to consecutive individuals to determine whether they will receive the active agent (a white packet) or a placebo (a red packet). As the clinic opens, the receptionist distributes all the white packets and then switches to the red packets until those also are gone. Although the receptionist did not know which color packet corresponded to which arm of the study (he being blinded), their conspicuous difference allowed him to distribute them nonrandomly. At first glance, randomization may appear to have been achieved, but due to the nonrandom sequence in which the packets were distributed, the study participants were not allocated at random.

With some luck the two groups may have contained similar distributions of sex, age, and other demographic factors despite a lack of randomization. However, they clearly do not contain equal numbers of individuals who preferred earlier appointments, compared with those who made later appointments. This seemingly subtle fact could mean that the experimental group (early arrivers, white packets) might as a group go to bed earlier than the control group (late appointments, red packets). This sort of unforeseen and inconspicuous, but possibly very important variable, is the type of bias against which proper randomization provides protection.

Suppose the researchers had a computer at the desk. As each individual arrived, the computer generated a random number. If this number were even, the individual would be assigned blindly to the treatment group, whereas if it were odd, the assignment would be to the control group. (The even-odd arrangement must not be known to the staff.) The time at which individuals arrived would make no difference; their assignments would be random. Alternatively, the researchers could have made all the packets the same color, shuffled them thoroughly, and sealed them. Then the receptionist would not have inadvertently "unrandomized" the distribution.

| Example | *Concealment*

To proceed with the previous example, assume that randomization was performed properly. A researcher who will not be involved in other aspects of the study (and who will not communicate with the other researchers) is assigned to screen the randomized candidates for eligibility in the study. As with most studies, certain exclusion criteria must be applied to ensure a safe and sound study (for example, use of other sleeping pills, concurrent diseases that also may affect sleep, or allergies to the drugs). As the researcher meets the enrollees, each provides her with the enrollment packet, after which she administers a questionnaire and screening exam. In reviewing the enrollment packet, she can ascertain to which group the individual has been assigned.

One exclusion criterion is the presence of underlying depression because the study drug is known to exacerbate depression. As she evaluates some enrollees who do not have histories of depression, she notes that several are quite haggard in appearance (very quiet and sad). Although the official criteria for depression are lacking, she senses that depression may be present nonetheless. She judges (perhaps subconsciously) that if such individuals have been assigned to the treatment group, exclusion from the study is in their best interests, lest the medication worsen their possible depression. If these individuals are in the control group, she has no such hesitation in admitting them into the study. The net result is that the control group is "stacked" with more depressed individuals than is the treatment group. Because depression is an important factor in cases of insomnia, this discrepancy may alter the results of the study, possibly making the drug "look" better than it is.

Had the original group assignment been concealed from the eligibility researcher, she would not have been able to exclude individuals selectively from one group.

| Example | *Blinding* |

In the sleeping pill study the researchers use a diary and interview technique to measure how long patients take to fall asleep after the lights are turned out. Human nature creates a desire to see the treatment work for many researchers, and positive research is more likely to be published, a concept known as *publication bias.* Blindness ensures that this eagerness to see a successful result does not affect the outcome of the study.

As the assessments are performed, one sleep-study researcher learns to which group the individuals are assigned through a paperwork mix-up. A patient he knows to be in the treatment group is asked, "You did fall asleep within 15 minutes of lights-out, correct?" whereas an individual known to be in the control group is asked, "How long after lights-out did it take you to fall asleep?" Even if the wording of the question were standardized, the manner in which it was asked might vary based on the unblinded researcher's awareness that the subject was or was not taking the active drug.

The two questions may elicit different responses, playing on the subject's desire to please the interviewer. In other cases, subjective interpretations of subtle radiologic or other test findings might be influenced similarly by the researcher's knowing the subject's treatment status.

**An exception to the blinding rule**  Blinding is not always possible, particularly in situations in which the treatment has obvious and unavoidable consequences (such as surgery) or universal side effects (alopecia from certain chemotherapeutic agents, for example).

Legend has it that the earliest studies on the efficacy of coronary artery bypass surgery compared the bypass group with a control group whose members underwent "sham" surgery, in which the skin was incised, the sternum split, the wounds sutured, and the participant returned to the room. Notwithstanding the admirable adherence to the concept of blinding, ethical justification for such a study would be difficult today. In any case, even this extreme approach resulted in the blinding of only one participant; the surgeon still knew which study participants underwent the actual bypass surgery.

To disqualify all studies of such treatments because they cannot be done blindly is unreasonable and unwise. In such cases, blinding should not be considered a primary criterion of validity. A better way to evaluate such studies is to examine how the researchers dealt with the issue. If the bulk of the outcomes measured appear to be physiologic, objective, and reasonably free from subjective influence (for example, mortality, creatinine levels), the lack of blinding may be acceptable. On the other hand, if the results deal with symptom diaries, reporting of subjective side effects, time until return to work, or even visual test result interpretations, the lack of blinding may prove a fatal flaw. As always the practitioner's clinical judgment is critical to this determination.

*The follow-through rule*   Were most subjects who entered the study followed to its conclusion and were they analyzed in the groups to which they were assigned originally?

This rule addresses the issue of continuity. Given the difficulties involved in the enrollment of individuals in almost any large clinical study, implied pressure exists to retain those who have enrolled. Thus if an individual does not tolerate a medication and discontinues it early in the course of the study, the researchers may be tempted to switch that participant to the control group. The goal is to track every single subject in the originally assigned group and analyze each subject as part of that group, whether or not the individual adhered to the protocol. This method usually is referred to as *intention-to-treat analysis,* the importance of which is appreciated best by example.

| *Example* |

A study is designed to compare surgical and medical treatment of acute appendicitis. Randomization and concealment are accomplished properly. Each group contains a random number of a total of 100 individuals. Of those assigned to the surgery group, two subjects die while awaiting surgery. The surgeons argue that these two participants should not be counted in the surgical results because they never even made it to surgery. The internists argue to the contrary; because the initial randomization presumably distributed the acuity of the individuals equally between the two groups, removal of two of the obviously most ill individuals from the surgical group will bias the study against medical treatment. Another surgeon even suggests that the two who died not only be removed from the surgical group but also actually be switched to the medical group because the only treatment they had received before they died was medical, not surgical.

If the "truth" were that both treatments carried a 2% mortality rate, removal of the two participants from the surgical group would have shown that group to have a 0% mortality; the medical group would have had its expected 2% mortality. If the individuals who died were switched to the medical group, the results would have been 0% and nearly 4%, respectively. In the end the closest approximation to the truth is to analyze the individuals in the group to which they were assigned originally.

Another scenario is that of 100 enrollees, 40 drop out before the conclusion of the study. The researcher may choose to analyze the remaining individuals, but without knowing the outcomes of the missing group, the conclusions would not be valid.

| *Example* |

Assume the sleeping-pill study has been well randomized with good concealment. The trial is underway. Over time, of the 80 individuals initially enrolled, 10 from each group of 40 fail to return for follow-up despite the best efforts of the researchers, leaving 30 participants in each group. One measure of treatment effect is sleep within 15 minutes, and the treatment group demonstrates a success rate of 67% (20 of 30 remaining participants), whereas the control group's success rate is 60% (18 of 30 remaining participants). The researchers conclude that the medication provided little benefit.

Information surfaces that 8 of the 10 control group dropouts did so because they were not feeling any better and did not find returning for follow-up care worth the trouble. (The other two were sleeping well.) Of the 10 treatment-group dropouts, 8 failed to return because they slept so well on the new medicine that they did not see the value in follow-up visits. (The other two still were sleeping poorly.) If we hypothetically put them back in the study, the success rate for the control group is 22 ÷ 40, or 55%, and the success rate for the treatment group is 28 ÷ 40, or 70%. These results would have made the medication appear much more effective than did the original results.

Stated in other terms, participants who drop out of studies may not do so randomly; important factors may be at work.

How much loss of follow-up is considered acceptable? The answer relates to the relationship between the dropout rate and the event rate (ER) of the outcome under study. The smaller the baseline ER or the dropout rate, the more tolerant the practitioner can be of deficient follow-up practices. The surest way to decide whether a dropout rate is acceptable is as follows:

- Note the number of dropouts, and assume that *all* such individuals did poorly (that is, failed to respond to the treatment).
- Plug the dropout numbers back into the results to determine whether the treatment still appears effective.

If the treatment does not appear effective based on the previously stated conditions, then the study's follow-up is insufficient. On the other hand, if the treatment appears effective even when all the dropouts are assumed to be "nonresponders," the dropout rate is clearly acceptable. However, assuming that all dropouts did poorly is a bit harsh for some studies; if the observed ERs in the remaining untreated participants are low, the practitioner may choose to presume something less than a total failure rate for the dropouts. In the end the issue is a judgment closely related to both the baseline ER in the control group and the actual percent of dropouts.

***Run-in periods*** At the other end of the follow-through rule is the concept of a *run-in period*. This term means that after randomization a study's participants are observed in the initial phase (run-in period) of treatment. If they cannot tolerate the treatment (or placebo), they may be either dropped from the study analysis or analyzed within their original groups. Dropping them from analysis measures *effectiveness* (whether the treatment *can* work in individuals who take it), whereas keeping them in their groups measures *efficacy* (real-world outcomes in the attempt to treat).

The harshest critics argue that researchers really want to know how the drug works in individuals who take it, not in those who do not. However, participants who fail to comply with the regimen may not be the same as those who do; in fact, perhaps they selectively represent those who are poor responders. Removing such participants may bias the results; if researchers discard them from the analysis, the remaining compliant individuals will represent only the better responders, and the treatment may appear better than it really is.

An additional point about the handling of noncompliant participants is that the clinician may find it useful to know that 50% of individuals fail to tolerate a drug, even if the drug is 90% effective in those who do tolerate it. Therefore reporting of compliance rates during a run-in period is helpful even when dropouts are not included in the final analysis. Thus readers must review treatment studies carefully to determine how intolerance was handled.

## Secondary Validity Criteria

Secondary validity criteria contribute to the soundness of a study to a variable extent. Practitioners must apply careful clinical judgment in determining whether the failure to meet any of these factors renders a given study invalid for the patient in question.

**Blinding**  The previous discussion noted that blinding is not always practical. When a practitioner believes that blinding is an important criterion and that its absence is a plausible cause of distorted results, it should be considered a primary "show-stopper" criterion. However, when blinding is impractical and the outcomes being measured are not necessarily highly dependent on the unblinded variable, the practitioner still may find the study valid. In such a case, blinding is considered a secondary criterion.

| *Example* |
|---|

An RCT of metoprolol in individuals with congestive heart failure found that the drug reduced mortality after 1 year by 3.7% (from 10.9% to 7.2%).[17] You know that this medication predictably slows the heart rate and suspect that the researchers might guess reliably which participants were in the experimental group through their slow pulse rates. Furthermore, you conclude that this inadvertent unblinding might affect clinical assessment but would be an unlikely cause of differences in death rates. Thus despite possible compromised blinding, you accept this imperfection as irrelevant to the conclusions of the study for mortality.

**Comparable Groups**  Were the groups similar at the outset of the study and treated similarly throughout the study, other than regarding the experimental treatment?

When the group size is sufficiently large, randomization usually balances incidental demographic and lifestyle differences between (or among) the groups. Practitioners should verify that randomization was adequate by specifically inspecting the data that compare such factors. (For some reason, this issue often is found in "Table 2" in treatment studies.) If differences do exist, the practitioner must use clinical knowledge and judgment to determine to what degree such discrepancies affect the patient in question.

For example, in a study on cardiovascular disease, the practitioner might not be comfortable with a substantial difference in tobacco use between the two groups. Age, gender, tobacco use, and diabetes mellitus are examples of factors that affect many diseases and often are addressed explicitly in the interpretation of clinical trials. Other factors are less universal but may be important in specific cases, such as prior replacement estrogen use in a study of osteoporosis.

The second aspect of the *comparable groups* criterion is that the groups, however similar at the outset, should be treated identically in terms of the study parameters. If one group is seen more often by the researchers; receives a different treatment, aside from the experimental treatment; or is exposed to possible risk or protective factors to a different extent than the other group, the study's validity is compromised. Practitioners should scan all treatment studies for signs of such discrepancies, although experience shows that sufficient detail often is unavailable to make such a judgment. Such deficiencies can occur occasionally, however, so practitioners should remain vigilant in their reviews.

| *Example* |

Researchers undertook a hypothetic study of upper respiratory infection rate and use of vitamin C. A group was assembled and a cross-over design implemented; each subject received placebo for 3 months, followed by vitamin C for 3 months. In this design each patient acted as his or her own "control" over time. Rates of upper respiratory symptoms were measured by use of a standardized survey. Careful scrutiny reveals that the study was initiated in June.

You recognize that the subjects received vitamin C for the 3 months in which an epidemiologically low incidence of upper respiratory infection occurred; the subjects received the placebo during the months in which the incidence was high. This observation may have distorted the data to make the treatment appear excessively effective. The outcomes may not reflect the treatment's true efficacy because the two phases of the study (treatment versus control) reflected different epidemiologic conditions that might have an important bearing on the outcome.

This discussion has covered the core concepts used to appraise a treatment study. First, applicability is assessed; if it is unacceptable, the study is disregarded. If applicability proves adequate, primary validity is addressed next, and if it is deemed unacceptable, the study is disregarded. If applicability and primary validity both are acceptable, secondary validity is assessed and a final judgment is made regarding the soundness of the evidence.

## Summary

This section addressed the importance of the careful appraisal of a research report in terms of its applicability to the patient and its validity in the accurate measurement of the phenomenon it claims to measure. The astute practitioner will approach this process systematically and efficiently before using the results for patient decision making.

Furthermore, assuming that the numeric results are valid, these numbers should be interpreted in light of their magnitude and confidence intervals. Statistically trivial or insignificant effects may not justify a given treatment.

# *Helping the Patient Decide*

## USING TREATMENT EVIDENCE IN MEDICAL DECISIONS

### The Master Decision Question

The Master Decision Question for treatments is as follows:

*Given the likelihood of improvements and risks of treatment, what is the impact of each outcome on the patient's quality of life and do the improvements outweigh the risks?*

This question is answered by calculation of a decision parameter known as the *action threshold (AT)*. The process is a form of risk-benefit analysis.

This chapter has discussed in detail how medical evidence is generated (study design) and reported (treatment parameters, such as ARR and NNT); it also has examined how to assess whether such studies are suitable for patients. Equipped with these parameters, readers can apply them to the basic task of medical management—making medical decisions. This task begins with an understanding of both sides of virtually every treatment—improvement in the target disease and harm from the treatment itself.

### Improvement

Improvement refers to desirable changes in the expected outcomes of a diseased patient brought about by the treatment. It is called *benefit* in many texts. Because *benefit* sometimes is used ambiguously and inconsistently, this book will not use the term.* Improvement can take several forms, as follows:

- Reduction in the likelihood of a symptom or symptoms
  *Example:* Antibiotics reduce the likelihood of death in patients treated for endocarditis.
- Reduction in the severity of a symptom
  *Example:* Analgesics reduce the intensity of self-reported pain after dental extraction by 50%.
- Increase in the frequency of a desirable outcome
  *Example:* Spironolactone increases the 2-year survival rate in congestive heart failure by 9%.
- Increase in the degree of a desirable outcome
  *Example:* When added to standard inhalers, ipratropium increases the improvement in pulmonary function tests by 7.3%.

To some extent, the way in which improvement is expressed is a semantic decision on the part of the researchers. In any case, when compared with those of an individual who does not take treatment, the overall outcomes of

---

*For the sake of comprehensiveness the correct definition of the word *benefit* is the same as this book's definition of *improvement*—the desirable changes in disease outcomes resulting from treatment. However, the concept of *net benefit* clouds the issue. *Net benefit* is the benefit minus harm due to treatment. Unfortunately, the two terms sometimes are confused and interchanged inappropriately. For clarity this book will ignore the term *net benefit* and use *improvement* instead of *benefit*.

the treated patient are expected to be superior on average. By definition, improvement applies solely to patients with disease. Patients without the disease who inadvertently receive treatment (a very common and often appropriate occurrence discussed later) have no likelihood of improvement from the treatment. The implication is that not all individuals diagnosed with a disease actually have the disease the physician suspects is present (the false positives).

## Harm

The dark side of treatment is described aptly as *harm*. This term refers to the side effects of the treatment distinct from the effects of the disease itself. Harm may take the form of a surgical complication, a drug reaction, or an increase in certain undesirable outcomes that could be caused by both the treatment and the disease.

To expand on this last point, imagine a disease with a mortality rate of 10%. An available treatment might improve this mortality by five absolute percentage points, down to 5%; however, the same treatment might itself cause death in 1% of individuals (even those without the disease). This harm offsets the mortality gain by 1%. True, a net gain of 4% remains, but the 1% death rate still is considered "harm" for this treatment. Harm, ideally, is determined through the study of healthy individuals (those who do not have the disease for which treatment is intended); it measures the undesired effects caused solely by the treatment. Realistically, many treatments are studied predominantly in diseased individuals for ethical and practical reasons, so the practitioner must compare control groups with the treated group, as discussed in the following section.

Why improvement is considered to apply only to diseased individuals is apparent, but why the practitioner would be interested in the harm of a treatment in individuals who do not even have the disease in question may create some confusion. The reason is that whenever uncertainty exists about a diagnosis, at least a small proportion of patients are treated in error; these individuals may have had false-positive test results, or testing may have been deemed unwarranted because of their high probability for disease. An example may help to clarify the meaning of the terms *harm* and *improvement* as this discussion has defined them thus far.

| Example |
| --- |

Studies have shown that the use of angiotensin-converting enzyme inhibitors, drugs commonly referred to as *ACE inhibitors,* reduces the death rate in certain groups of individuals with congestive heart failure from approximately 22% to approximately 16% over several months.[6] Reports have stated that approximately 12% of individuals taking the ACE inhibitor enalapril developed substantial side effects, such as low blood pressure, kidney failure, or major allergic reactions requiring medical treatment and discontinuation of the drug (these figures being in excess of their rates with placebo).[15] This heart-failure population was especially vulnerable to the side effects, compared with the general population.

The improvement in the previous example is the decreased mortality rate, impressive at 6% ARR over a few months. The harm is the 12% incidence of side effects. Although the risk of harm likely would not dissuade the practitioner from prescribing this drug to appropriate patients, that physician certainly would not want to expose patients to this drug if the benefit were not great.

To express how "good" or "bad" a treatment is, the practitioner must be able to describe harm and improvement in quantitative terms. Once that task is complete, the practitioner then (1) can decide whether a treatment is worthwhile and (2) compare one treatment with another in a quantitative manner. The following section discusses this technique.

## The Action Threshold

### Describing the Harm and Improvement of a Treatment in Evidence-Based Terms
This section introduces the reader to the term *action threshold (AT)*, which is a single number incorporating all components necessary to quantify the harm and improvements attributable to a treatment. Intellectually powerful and numerically simple, the AT is a sophisticated concept that can be mastered easily.

The AT is essentially a refinement of the traditional expression known as *risk-benefit ratio*. Practitioners weigh the advantages and disadvantages of treatments all the time, but rarely quantitatively. Explicit use of the AT can provide greater consistency in such judgments. In addition, the patient's values receive more rigorous attention, and the practitioner can make trustworthy comparisons between two or more treatment options. In essence the AT is a score reflecting how "wise" a treatment is for a specific patient.

The AT is represented on a numeric scale in which *lower* scores represent *better* treatments. It is unitless and always positive. It is meaningful primarily as a relative score compared with other treatments or the option of "no treatment." The AT is designed for use within a specific disease-treatment scenario and is not useful outside that scenario. No specific AT can be assigned generically to a given treatment-disease diad; the threshold changes for every patient and every scenario.

## The Action Threshold as a Logical Paradigm

The following sections deal with the calculations needed to derive an AT. However, the reader may find an understanding of the concept as a logical paradigm useful. Consider the following examples.

Imagine a disease that is universally fatal. Imagine a treatment that is completely curative in all individuals with the dreadful disease, trivial to undergo, and free of cost and has absolutely no side effects or risks. Clearly, if you had this disease, you would proceed at once with treatment. In fact, if you were only 50% confident you had the disease, you would seek treatment promptly, and so on down to virtually any suspicion of disease. Figure 3.2, *A*, depicts this scenario.

Now consider the previous scenario—but with one important alteration; the treatment in question causes fatality in 10% of individuals who take it. Certain that you had the disease, you likely still would choose treatment but worry more about its risks. On the other hand, if you were faced with only a 10% chance of having the disease, undergoing treatment would be a neutral decision; without treatment, you would die 10% of the time (that is, a 10% chance of having the universally fatal illness), and with treatment, you would not die of the disease but would have a 10% chance of dying from the treatment itself. Figure 3.2, *B*, depicts this situation.

Next, consider the scenario with a 20% chance that you have illness. Without treatment the death risk from disease is 20%. With treatment, you take no risk of dying from the disease but encounter a 10% chance of dying from the illness. The only rational conclusion is to take the treatment (10% mortality) because not doing so exposes you to a higher risk of death (20% mortality from disease). A similar but converse conclusion would result if you had a 1% chance of having the disease; you likely would forego treatment, considering it the riskier decision.

In the example, 10% corresponds to the AT for this disease-treatment diad. Neither treatment decision would yield a *certain* outcome, but, given the odds the practitioner and patient can be certain which decision is correct.* Readers may recognize already that most real-world scenarios involve risks and improvements far less clear than those provided in the previous examples.

## The Action Threshold from the Patient's Perspective

The discussion now progresses to the nonquantitative implications of ATs from the patient perspective. Faced with the likelihood of a given disease, the pa-

---

*If the chance a patient has the disease is *exactly* the same as the AT, both decisions can mean the same risk of death. The patient has little reason to take the treatment in such a case. In practice, close calls similar to this situation generally warrant further testing, if possible.

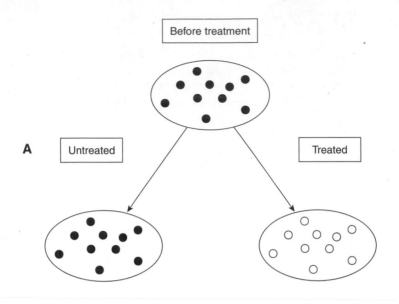

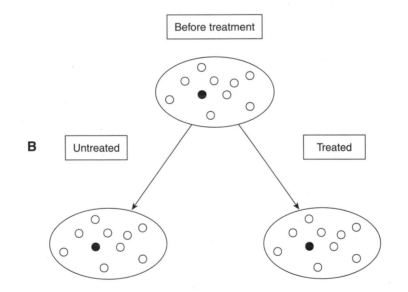

**Figure 3.2    A,** Black circles indicate anticipated deaths; white circles indicate cures. In this case, all patients have the disease, and the treatment is uniformly curative and has no side effects. Treatment is the only logical choice if the initial suspicion of disease is greater than 0. **B,** Introduction of a risk to the treatment decision. The decision becomes a toss-up. Thus any pretreatment likelihood of disease greater than 10% favors the treatment decision, whereas a likelihood less than 10% favors no treatment.

**TABLE 3.2**

Factors Considered in Decision Analysis

| Factor | Comments |
| --- | --- |
| Natural course of current illness and health | What will happen if I do not take treatment? Is this disease self-limiting or chronic? |
| Likelihood that treatment will improve symptoms and prognosis | Is the treatment sure-fire? Does it benefit only a small proportion of patients? |
| Importance placed on improvements the treatment might bring* | If I do not find the improvements very important, will I benefit from taking treatment? |
| Likelihood of side effects | Are side effects highly likely or rare? |
| Intensity of side effects* | If I experience the side effect, will I accept it as simple bad luck? |
| Other issues* | How do the cost, discomfort, disability, and preferences of friends and loved ones factor into my decision? |

*Indicates individual or subjective factors.

tient must decide whether to accept a treatment. To do so that patient must consider many factors (Table 3.2).

The tradition in medicine is for the physician to bundle all these factors into a sound "intuition" and then advise the patient accordingly. The decision is indeed obvious in many cases to most physicians, but a surprisingly high occurrence of situations arise in which the physician should question this approach.

Of the elements listed in Table 3.2, some are quantitative parameters that usually can be determined through the tools of EBM; others are subjective and individual. To impose a decision on a patient without attending to the crucial subjective elements is ill-advised of the physician; to make presumptions about patients based on personal feelings (rather than those of the patient) is not much better.

The AT accounts for all elements in decision making—subjective and objective. It is not a perfect tool and cannot account for all the human and intangible subtleties of a decision; however, it is a great improvement over whatever is second best as a tool used to assess treatments. For the patient the AT allows for the synthesis of each objective and subjective factor into a single numeric score.

**Numeric Parameters of the Action Threshold**  By now the reader should have a qualitative sense of what the AT represents. To be useful in decision making, the AT also must have a quantitative definition. A simplified mathematic representation of the AT is as follows:

$$AT = \frac{harm}{improvement}$$

Although the formula is incomplete (expanded in the following section), what is clear is that the greater the improvement, the *lower* the AT; conversely, the greater the harm, the *higher* the AT.

### How to Interpret Action Threshold Values

***An action threshold greater than 1*** An AT greater than 1 means that the treatment makes no sense for the patient, even if it is curative in all cases. Treatment in such cases is illogical.

> *Absurd example:* Amputation above the knee cures all cases of ingrown toenail.
>
> *Not-so-absurd conclusion:* The AT does not simply reflect the efficacy of the treatment but rather reflects its efficacy *relative to its harm* in the context of the disease at hand.

Thus a single treatment may have numerous ATs, depending on the disease it aims to treat (for example, amputation for gangrene instead of ingrown toenail). As mentioned previously, the AT is only meaningful for comparisons and decisions *within the treatment-disease diad* for the patient at hand. Comparing absolute ATs across different scenarios is not useful.

***A very high action threshold (but less than 1)*** This treatment's improvements and harm tip only slightly in favor of the option to proceed with the treatment.

> *Example:* Radiation and chemotherapy are available for most metastatic cancers. The treatment is grueling and has very significant risks, the disease often responds in a limited way, and the decision whether to treat is often marginal and personal. You would not proceed with treatment without a very high level of confidence about the diagnosis, with full expectation that side effects will occur.

***A very low action threshold*** When the AT is quite low, the patient may consider taking the treatment even though that patient is uncertain about the presence of the disease because the risk is low and/or the improvements (if the patient does have the disease) are so clear.

> *Example:* You excise a mildly "suspicious" mole even though the risk of eventual malignancy may be quite low because the treatment is safe. On the other hand, the improbable melanoma could be more dangerous.

**The Action Threshold as a Diagnostic Test Target** The previous interpretations of AT refer to situations in which the practitioner is confident about the diagnosis and is determining whether treatment is the correct decision. In addition, the AT has another extremely useful interpretation in situations in which the diagnosis is uncertain; the AT corresponds to the diagnostic probability above which treatment is the best decision for the patient and below which treatment is not the best decision. For example, in the diagnosis of group A β-hemolytic strep throat, the usual tests virtually never allow the physician to achieve 100% confidence (because of false-positive and false-negative results). The AT of penicillin for this condition may work out to 0.4; thus if the physician's diagnostic confidence is 40% or higher, treatment is the best decision; the physician may not need to test to a level higher. (This concept will be developed more fully in the Diagnosis chapter.)

## Calculating the Action Threshold

*Harm and improvement—by the numbers* The previous discussion demonstrated that the AT may be expressed as the ratio of harm to improvement. This expression requires the quantitative expression of each term. In turn, both harm and improvement have two separate components—the frequency (probability) of the outcome in question* and its subjective importance, or *impact*. Both parts are expressed on the 0-to-1 scale:

$$\text{Harm} = \text{frequency} \times \text{impact (harmful outcomes)}$$

and

$$\text{Improvement} = \text{frequency} \times \text{impact (desired outcomes)}$$

*Frequency* With the tools discussed previously, most practitioners can determine quickly how frequently a side effect will occur based on valid and appropriate evidence. Often this evidence boils down to one or two side effects of importance.

| Example |
| --- |

> In a study of donepezil in elderly individuals for the treatment of Alzheimer's disease, nausea or diarrhea occurred in 11% of the placebo group versus 35% of the group treated with 10 mg of the drug daily, a statistically important difference.[23] The frequency of these side effects due to the drug thus is 35% minus 11%, or 24%.

*Impact* The term *impact* refers to the personal, subjective importance of a given outcome to the patient. It is expressed as a number from 0 to 1. When assigning an impact score to an outcome, the patient does not focus on whether the outcome is good, bad, or intermediate; a horrid outcome would have a very strong impact and thus probably be assigned a very high impact score. By the same token a wonderful, life-changing improvement also would have a major impact and receive a high impact score. What matters is how

---

*The frequency of side effects refers to outcomes attributable to the treatment itself (that is, the difference between the treated group and the control group). If 80% of urinary infections improve spontaneously within 5 days and 94% do so with treatment, the improvement frequency is not 80%, but 94% *minus* 80%, or 14%.

profoundly it affects the patient's quality of life. The "goodness" or "badness" is addressed in the equation by virtue of the outcome being considered as "harm" versus "improvement." Its score simply reflects its power to affect the patient's quality of life.

Although consideration of a very common side effect as "worse" than a rare one is natural, the subjective component (that is, the "worse" part) should be reserved for the quality of the side effect itself. In other words, explicit separation of frequency from impact is important. In assigning impact scores the practitioner assumes that the patient would experience the particular outcome in question. That the outcome occurs in only 1% of patients is irrelevant; practitioners should score each outcome as though the patient were the 1 in 100 who *would be* affected. Human nature tends to lead individuals to overestimate the impact of common occurrences and underestimate that of rare occurrences. Actually the fact that the occurrence is rare or common should not factor into the impact estimate; frequency is accounted for elsewhere in the AT equation.

No "right" or "wrong" score for a given impact actually exists. The score is strictly personal and depends on a host of contextual issues. However, the practitioner often can sense when a patient seems to attribute an unexpected or even irrational impact to an outcome. This instance may be due to misunderstanding, previously unidentified social or psychologic factors, or other issues that must be clarified and discussed. Although the practitioner should not presume to know the patient's thoughts and feelings when discussing impacts, objectively identifying and clarifying those occasions in which such inappropriate assignations seem to occur is useful.

> *An aside:* Readers who have read elsewhere about the quantification of patient opinions and values regarding clinical outcomes have encountered the word *utilities.* Utilities are similar to impacts except that they are scalar. Worse outcomes always are assigned lower utilities than are better outcomes. A utility of 1 is the best case, and a utility of 0 is the worst case. Such a system is necessary for the traditional calculation of decision trees and influence diagrams, both of which are advanced tools for decision analysis. However, when used for simple and practical day-to-day decision making, this scalar property makes such tools cumbersome. The reader is advised to be aware of the distinction. This book will use the impact approach, which is easier to understand and to learn. Readers who wish to pursue more advanced topics in decision analysis should find that the concept of utilities becomes clear quite readily after they understand impacts.

## Assigning Impacts

Although subjective, impacts can be described with a numeric scale, much the way patients are asked to rate pain on a scale from 0 to 10. Several methods are available.

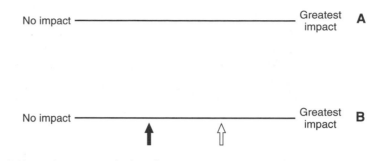

**Figure 3.3** **A,** Linear placement method used to estimate impact scores. A line represents the spectrum of impact a given outcome might have on the patient's quality of life. **B,** Patient-drawn arrows correspond to their estimated impacts for corrected vision (*black arrow*) and monocular blindness (*white arrow*).

**Method 1: Linear Placement** This method involves the drawing of a literal or imaginary vertical or horizontal line. Conventionally, the left or bottom of the line represents 0, and the right or top represents 1. The practitioner simply should request the patient to position each relevant outcome somewhere on the line corresponding to its impact by working through the harmful outcomes first and then proceeding to the desirable outcomes for clarity. The advantage of explicit placement of these outcomes is that it combines the cognitive assessment with a visual layout.

> *Example*

A patient is assessing the impact of blindness in one eye as a complication of surgery for correction of visual acuity. The two impacts under consideration are as follows:

- Monocular blindness (a side effect of surgery)
- Markedly reduced need for corrective lenses to correct visual acuity (an improvement expected from surgery)

You draw a line similar to the one in Figure 3.3, *A,* and ask the patient to place a mark or arrow on that line corresponding to the impact of each outcome. In so doing, you define the concept of impact for the patient. One description might be as follows:

*"This line represents just how powerfully this outcome would affect the quality of your life. This is a personal judgment, and there are no right or wrong answers. One at a time, we will assume you experience each outcome. Draw a mark on the line that reflects the impact of each outcome. Note that both good and bad events can have high or low impacts. We are interested in how powerful the impact is, not how good or bad it is."*

The practitioner may want to illustrate the technique with an unrelated example, taking care to show, for example, how death and a life saved likely would have the same impact. In addition, the practitioner should ensure that the patient does not include the *likelihood* of an outcome in this exercise; instead the patient must assume the outcome actually has occurred.

Figure 3.3 illustrates how the patient may respond to this exercise. Figure 3.3, *B*, shows the arrows drawn at approximately 0.33 and 0.66 (on a scale of 1). Under the assumption that this placement at least seems plausible, the practitioner would accept the scores as rational and consistent* and consider using the values in the AT calculation. The linear placement method has both advantages and disadvantages, as follows:

*Advantages*
- Is relatively simple to understand and perform
- Allows for head-to-head simultaneous comparisons of all outcomes

*Disadvantages*
- Can be confusing
- Demonstrates a lower statistical reliability over time, compared with other tools

Although no sound "outcome" evidence validates this tool in the assessment of impacts, experience has shown that its simplicity often makes it a good choice. With experience, each practitioner can quickly develop clear, neutral, and consistent ways to present the scenarios to patients verbally and graphically. A side benefit is that the exercise itself often elicits questions and thoughts about the clinical decision that can enhance the patient's understanding of the medical and social ramifications of treatment options.

**Method 2: Verbal Estimation** A patient may lack the quantitative skills or experience to participate in the linear placement exercise. The practitioner then may use purely verbal descriptions to elicit the same information. In such cases the practitioner runs the risk of making incorrect assumptions about the patient's true intentions and feelings. Following a structured approach should reduce such occurrences.

> | *Example* |

You explicitly summarize a patient's current health state. For example, you may phrase a patient's condition as follows:

*"Mr. Smith, you currently have very poor vision and require eyeglasses for both reading and distant vision. You need to either wear bifocals, which you find unpleasant, or carry two pairs of glasses, which you interchange often throughout the day. Is that a fair summary?"*

---

*In the example (Figure 3.3, *B*) the patient estimated the impact of monocular blindness as greater than that of corrected vision. This factor does not necessarily mean that the treatment in question is irrational because the *frequency* of occurrence for blindness is so much lower than that for corrected vision. This example illustrates the importance of the consideration of frequency and impact as discrete elements.

Next, you describe the harmful outcome in the following similar way:

*"Imagine that the operation leaves you with no vision at all in your left eye. You would still require glasses for your right eye. With no vision in the left eye, you would experience decreased ability to see on the left side and some loss of depth perception. Your visual skills for athletic and other activities requiring keen vision would be reduced permanently. You would lose the safety of having both eyes, a significant fact if you later develop problems with your right eye."*

You then ask this patient the following question:

*"Compared with how things are right now, how large an impact would losing the vision in your left eye have on the quality of your life?"*

If you leave the question at that, you are likely to hear the patient respond that such a situation would be awful. You must quantify the query by adding a qualifying phrase such as the following:

*"Would this vision loss be a very severe impact, a moderate impact, or a mild impact?"*

However, you can change the wording to fit the scenario. You might even be able to use the following question, with minor modification:

*"On a scale of 0 to 5, where 5 is the worst you can imagine (such as death), how would you rate the impact of losing vision in one eye?"*

You next perform an analogous task for the improvements likely to be brought about by corrective surgery. For example, you might say the following:

*"Mr. Smith, we just summarized your current vision status. Imagine now that surgery is successful. Although you still may need reading glasses for small print or dim surroundings, you should be able to perform most other tasks without the need for glasses or contact lenses. How much of an impact would this improvement have on your overall quality of life—extreme, moderate, or mild?"*

Alternatively, you might use a similar scale to that used previously:

*"On a scale of 0 to 5, where 5 is the best impact you can imagine (for example, perfect vision without glasses), how would you rate the impact of successful surgery on the quality of your life?"*

Experienced physicians can recognize immediately that nearly every clinical scenario requires significant improvisation. The essential ingredient is to keep the descriptions neutral in tone, clinically accurate, and nonjudgmental in their wording; sneaking in a quantitative "Likert-like" scale (for example, 0 to 5) as in the previous example can be useful. This common method is applicable universally because almost all unimpaired patients can provide a general sense of their values surrounding a given outcome. The method has not been (and perhaps cannot be) validated statistically, but its usefulness seems apparent in comparison with the customary total absence of attention that patient values often receive in the decision process.

The two methods of impact estimation discussed in the following sections are more systematic and have been used formally in decision analysis. Practitioners who can achieve comfort with these methods should use them preferentially, at least in selected situations (that is, when time, patient ability, or stakes warrant).

**Method 3: Comparing Two Impacts: Time Trade-Off**   Because the impact of harm and improvement are compared ultimately as a *ratio* in the AT equation (harm ÷ improvement), their absolute numbers are not critical if their ratio accurately reflects the patient's values. For this reason, practitioners who can compare the two clearly may be able to work around the difficulty of assigning a specific numeric value to either one. In other words, if one impact is twice as strong as the other, whether their respective scores are 0.2 and 0.4, 0.1 and 0.2, or 0.5 and 1 is irrelevant; the ratio remains unchanged. Time trade-off is a method that takes advantage of this fact.

The time trade-off method is based on the presumption that life in a healthy state is valued more highly than life in a less healthy state; thus sacrificing some amount of life expectancy in poor health may be worthwhile in return for better health and a shorter life span. This method measures the trade-off of quantity for quality. Thus the time trade-off method often is a better fit for patients with long-term health problems than for those in short-term states.

| Example |
|---------|

> Paul has suffered a stroke that has left him weak in the right arm and leg. He cannot get out of bed without assistance and must use a wheelchair. He was in perfect health before the onset of his stroke. His life expectancy is 10 years in his current state. In a philosophic moment, he muses that he would give up 8 years of his remaining life gladly to live just 2 years in his previously unimpaired state of health.

This example illustrates that for serious impairments, life span and life quality form an intimate bond in terms of patient values and judgments. The example shows that the 10-year life expectancy in poor health should be "quality-adjusted" downward to equate to 2 years in good health. The term *quality-adjusted life years (QALY)* is used often in cost-benefit analyses but is relevant in this setting as well.

When using the time trade-off method for impact estimation, the physician compares the various possible outcomes to the independent outcome of the patient's baseline, premorbid health. The physician then asks the patient to estimate how many years of baseline health would be acceptable in return for a fixed period of time with the current imperfect health state. The generic time trade-off question as it applies to undesirable outcomes is as follows:

> How many [*a plausible time period*] in [*the premorbid baseline health*] would you accept in exchange for living [*a plausible time period*] with [*the disease state or side effect in question*]?

Because this example is generic, the bracketed text must be tailored to the individual scenario. The patient will respond presumably with some period of time less than 10 years. (If not, the patient has not understood the question.) The impact of this scenario in question would be the proportion by which the patient's response differs from 10, or (10 − response) ÷ 10. In the previous example the stroke patient estimated that 2 years in perfect health would be his trade-off against 10 years with hemiparesis. Thus 8 of 10 years are worth sacrificing to him, an impact of 8 ÷ 10, or 0.8. Substituting an interval other than 10 requires replacement of 10 in the equation with the new value.

The following examples illustrate how variations on this technique can apply to different situations. The variable data are tailored to fit the different medical realities, as follows:

---

**Examples**

> ***Scenario:*** Impact of allergic rhinitis in an otherwise healthy young patient
> *Trade-off:* How many years free of nasal symptoms would you accept in return for living another 40 years with your current runny nose and nasal congestion?
> *Typical response:* 39.9 years
> *Interpretation:* The impact of allergic rhinitis based on this response is (40 − 39.9) ÷ 40, or 0.003, on a scale of 0 to 1. The impact is trivial, but if the harm of treatment were sufficiently low, the treatment may remain a viable option.
> *Comment:* This technique stretches the limits of plausibility when the outcomes in question are mild or trivial; it works best for serious impairments.

> ***Scenario:*** Impact of moderate asthma in an otherwise healthy young patient
> *Trade-off:* How many years completely free of asthma would you accept in return for living another 40 years with your current shortness of breath, cough, and ongoing medication requirements?
> *Typical response:* 30 years
> *Interpretation:* The impact of asthma based on this scenario is (40 − 30) ÷ 40, or 0.25, on a scale of 0 to 1.

> ***Scenario:*** Impact of asthma treatment (side effects)
> *Trade-off:* How many years completely free of side effects would you accept in return for living another 40 years with mild tremor, the need to use an inhaler 4 times daily, and twice yearly courses of prednisone-induced swelling and sleeplessness?
> *Typical response:* 36 years
> *Interpretation:* The impact of drugs based on this case is (40 − 36) ÷ 40, or 0.1, on a scale of 0 to 1.

> ***Scenario:*** Impact of diabetes on a 50-year-old patient
> *Trade-off:* How many years of life free of diabetes would you accept in return for living another 20 years with your current need for insulin, occasional hypoglycemic symptoms, poor vision, and intermittent burning feet?

*Typical response:* 15 years

*Interpretation:* The impact of diabetes for this patient is $(20 - 15) \div 20$, or 0.25, on a scale of 0 to 1.

**Method 4: Bracketing** Time trade-off is sometimes awkward to use with short-term issues because few patients are willing to sacrifice *any* life expectancy to prevent, for example, 3 days of diarrhea right now. However, trade-offs can be used to *compare* two short-term outcomes. Once the practitioner knows how the outcomes compare in proportion to one another, comparably proportionate impacts can be assigned in the AT calculation. (The absolute impact scores are irrelevant; the importance lies in their *ratio*.)

Following are the steps involved in the impact-comparison technique and some additional examples to help readers become familiar with the technique:

- Phrase the disease symptoms and side effects in neutral terms, expressing both as undesirable outcomes.
- Ask the patient to compare living with each symptom for a reasonable amount of time to determine which symptom the patient considers "better" (the one the patient would rather tolerate).
- Gradually reiterate the comparison, holding the interval for the "worse" outcome stable while shortening the interval for the "better" outcome. At some point the comparably brief exposure to the better outcome should become the patient's preferred scenario.
- Gradually lengthen the interval for the better outcome until the choice becomes a toss-up.
- The two intervals now reflect the impacts for the AT. Convert calculations to numbers from 0 to 1 (for example, 5 days versus 7 days converting to 0.5 versus 0.7; 8 months to 15 months converting to 0.4 to 0.75) and always assign the *smaller* number to the *better* outcome in your original scenario.

> ### Examples

Consider the use of antibiotics to treat acute sinusitis. Assume that antibiotics can cause an itchy rash for 3 days* and that successful treatment shortens the duration of sinus pain by 3 days. The goal is to estimate relative impacts for these two outcomes (rash and sinus pain), as follows:
- Phrase both outcomes in undesirable terms—sinus pain and itchy rash.
- Find out which outcome the patient considers "better," possibly by asking if the patient had to experience one outcome for 3 days, which would that patient choose. The preferred outcome becomes the variable in the time trade-off. For now, assume that the patient would rather live with the rash.

---

*Some readers may wonder about the occasional anaphylactic reaction to antibiotics. Aside from a desire to keep the example straightforward, such severe reactions are notably so rare (for example, 1:200,000) that they almost never affect the ultimate decision. In scenarios in which the risk is less than 1:10,000 or so, this risk approaches the risk that an individual may die in such a rare natural event as an automobile accident. Society assumes that such risk is an acceptable trade-off in the context of daily life.

- State the possible outcomes.

*Trade-off:* If you had to live for 5 days with sinus pain or 6 days with the rash alone, which would you choose?
*Typical response:* Rash

- Reword the question to make the answer a bit harder for the patient; change the numbers to make the choice a bit more difficult.

*Trade-off:* If you had to live for 5 days with sinus pain alone or 10 days with the rash alone, which would you choose?
*Typical response:* Sinus pain

- Because the boundary at which the patient would reverse the decision (somewhere between 6 and 10 days) has been crossed, once again adjust the numbers to make the decision more difficult.

*Trade-off:* If you had to live 5 days with sinus pain alone or 7 days with the rash alone, which would you choose?
*Typical response:* A "toss-up"

In the previous example the toss-up ratio of 5:7 becomes the impact ratio. It corresponds to the impact of the better outcome, and the impact of the worse outcome is assigned a value of 1.

The example details the following necessary steps used to compare the impact of two outcomes:

1. Statement of both as undesirable
2. Determination of which is worse
3. Trade-off through adjustment of the duration of the better outcome against a fixed duration of the worse until a toss-up is achieved
4. Expression of the resulting ratio as numbers between 0 and 1
5. Plugging of those values into the AT equation

Yet another example may help reinforce the technique, this time in the form of a dialogue between patient and physician. (Comments in parentheses refer to the previously mentioned steps.)

Examples

*Physician:* We need to decide whether to treat your painful diabetic neuropathy with amitriptyline. If we do not treat it, assume that your painful feet will remain unchanged for the next 6 months. If we treat it, your pain probably will be reduced but you will experience moderate fatigue. It is a trade-off
First, assuming you had only one symptom, tell me whether you would rather live with moderate fatigue for the next 6 months or instead with your current foot pain for 6 months? (Determine which of the two choices is worse.)
*Patient:* Fatigue (Fatigue is better; foot pain is worse.)

*Physician:* Suppose now that you had a choice—3 months of foot pain or 6 months of fatigue. Which would you prefer? (Begin adjusting to find out where the patient's threshold is.)

*Patient:* Foot pain (Foot pain is bad but not worth the trade-off for an extra 3 months of fatigue.)

*Physician:* Suppose you had to choose between 3 months of foot pain and 5 months of fatigue. (Make the decision more difficult.)

*Patient:* That's too close to call; one is as bad as the other. (Bingo; these are the toss-up values—3 versus 5 months.)

*Conclusion:* The ratio of 3 months to 5 months is 0.6:1. Fatigue assumes a relative impact of 0.6 (the smaller value being assigned to the better outcome), whereas foot pain receives a value of 1.

To complete the example, certain assumptions must be made, as follows:
- The frequency of fatigue with amitriptyline is 40%.
- Foot pain is a certainty without treatment.
- Treatment is 75% effective.

Both harm and improvement are products of their respective frequency and impact scores, as in the following equation:

$$\frac{\text{Harm} = 0.4 \times 0.6 = 0.24}{\text{Improvement} = 0.75 \times 1 = 0.75}$$

The AT for this example is 0.32. This value is interpreted to support a decision to treat (AT under 1) unless alternative treatments with even lower ATs are present. Readers can repeat the decision analysis, assuming that the treatment was only effective 25% of the time rather than 75% to emphasize the necessity of considerations of frequency and impact in all decisions.

Applying the time trade-off method with or without bracketing can be adapted to many clinical scenarios. To improvise such scenarios requires practice, but the time trade-off provides a sturdy means to elicit patient values that are unable to be quantified more directly.

## A Concession to Practicality

Although line drawing and creation of time trade-off scenarios have clear value in the eliciting of patient values and preferences, most physicians, in the course of a busy clinical practice, cannot perform these procedures regularly. In fact, many medical decisions regarding treatment are straightforward and do not require a formal approach. Physicians who find themselves seeking shortcuts to deal with such practicalities at least can calculate a rough AT by substituting self-determined sensible impact scores derived by placing themselves in the mindsets of their patients (considering age, gender, health, and social setting).

Although to what extent the physician can presume accurately how the patient feels about a given outcome is questionable, this approach forces the physician to consider explicitly all the relevant issues at hand. The role-playing approach may seem presumptuous, but when tempered by sensitivity and thoughtfulness, it likely will serve the patient better than a purely intuitive decision. Physicians may be surprised how often their initial reactions come under scrutiny when they analyze it from the patient's view.

> *Example*

A mildly demented and moderately debilitated 72-year-old man must decide whether to undergo chemotherapy for metastatic colon cancer. You know that the patient accepts death in the near future and has planned appropriately. His family seems to have adjusted well to his plight. The chemotherapy reportedly increases survival in about 20% of patients similar to this man from 4 months to 1 year. The toxicity rate for diarrhea is 38%, whereas 37% of individuals studied experienced serious skin or mucosal lesions.[2] He and the family ask you whether chemotherapy is wise.

You estimate the impact of prolonged life from 4 months to 1 year as very meaningful, with an impact of 0.67.* You judge the impact of severe diarrhea or skin and mucosal lesions as important to the quality of his remaining life but less so than prolonged survival, and you assign these side effects an impact of 0.3. Using these estimates, you construct the AT equation as follows:

$$\frac{\text{Harm} = 0.75 \times 0.3 = 0.23}{\text{Improvement} = 0.2 \times 0.67 = 0.13}$$

$$\text{AT} = \frac{0.23}{0.13} = 1.8 \text{ (unacceptable result)}$$

Because the AT is greater than 1, chemotherapy is not advisable under the conditions stated in the previous example. The example did not use a linear placement model or time trade-off to estimate the impacts, but such impacts were addressed explicitly in the practitioner's thinking.

To emphasize just how important individual factors and values are (and therefore how important use of the *patient's* impacts rather than the practitioner's), the previous scenario can be used with one change. The patient's youngest daughter is expecting her first child in 8 months, and this milestone is extremely important to the patient so that he can die in peace. The impact of

---

*The impact of prolonged life can be tricky, but assignation of a value proportional to the prolongation divided by the optimum survival period is reasonable. In this case the improvement is from 4 months to 1 year, or 8 months. The optimum survival period Is 1 year, and thus the impact is $8 \div 12$, or 0.67 if the optimum survival period were 36 months, the impact of survival from 4 months to 36 months would be $32 \div 36$, for an impact of 0.89. For quality-of-life outcomes, as opposed to survival outcomes, the practitioner generally estimates the impact as if the outcomes were present for whatever period of time the treatment would be administered, or for the rest of the patient's life if the outcomes cause permanent impairment.

prolonged survival by 8 months now is much higher, and the important survival number might be 5 months rather than 8, thereby raising its likelihood;
the decision to take chemotherapy might change.

Readers should see clearly now that impacts form a core component of treatment decision making. Explicit incorporation of impacts into treatment decisions
may be time consuming, but failure to do so places patients' interests at risk.

**Action Threshold: Handling Scenarios with Numerous Outcomes** Until
now, this chapter's discussion has considered only the impact and frequency
of a single side effect compared to a single improvement. In clinical medicine,
physicians sometimes are faced with many potential side effects and
improvements. The proper method used to deal with these choices is an
extension of the method discussed previously and involves the calculation of
a *weighted average* for the impacts of all of the important outcomes.

For example, a treatment has three important side effects, and the physician
wants to consider them all in the calculation. For each separate outcome the
physician retrieves a likelihood of occurrence and then an impact estimation.
The following table illustrates this process, listing three side effects from a single treatment, with the aggregate harm calculated as the sum of the probability-
impact product of all the rows:

| Outcome | Probability | Impact | Product |
|---------|-------------|--------|---------|
| Itchy rash | 0.2 | 0.1 | 0.02 |
| Severe headache | 0.1 | 0.3 | 0.03 |
| Vomiting | 0.1 | 0.3 | 0.03 |
| **Sum** | | | 0.08 |

The rightmost column displays the product of the probability and impact
for each row. Multiple outcomes all are listed, and the product of each row is
added to produce one final sum. In this case the sum is 0.08, which would be
considered the aggregate *harm* of the weighted side effects.

The procedure for the improvements of treatment A now is repeated, with
the assumption that the treatment also has two major improvements, and the
aggregate improvement is calculated as shown in the following table:

| Outcome | Probability | Impact | Product |
|---------|-------------|--------|---------|
| Pain resolved | 0.7 | 0.5 | 0.35 |
| Fatigue improved | 0.5 | 0.2 | 0.1 |
| **Sum** | | | 0.45 |

By use of the "sum of the products" as the numerator and denominator, the AT is estimated as 0.08 ÷ 0.45, or 0.18. Under the assumption that the diagnosis was certain, the AT can be interpreted to favor treatment over no treatment.

*A Caution:* This method of handling multiple outcomes makes presumptions that may not always apply to all cases. It assumes that the outcomes in each table are mutually exclusive. Although this assumption is not typically so (both headache and rash being possible in the same patient), the weighting tends to mathematically "smooth out" such occurrences. Still, situations exist in which the combined frequencies of numerous side effects exceed 100%. Because such a percentage is not possible, the implication is that some patients will experience multiple side effects. At least in theory this practice can lead to a combined impact greater than 1, in which case the mathematic model fails. (I have yet to encounter such a scenario in actual practice.) The methodologic alternatives used to deal with such situations are beyond the scope of this book but rarely are relevant to most readers.

## Legitimacy of the Action Threshold in Medical Decision Making

Few observers would argue with the mathematic legitimacy of the use of the AT approach to decision making about treatments. If the numbers used in the calculation are based on sound evidence and the impacts truly reflect the patient's values, the conclusions are axiomatic.[21] As many business professionals discovered, the use of risk, expenses, and revenue (analogous to frequency, harm, and improvement) allows for the accurate calculation of "break-even point."

However, impacts are not dollars, and the tools used to elicit them are far from precise and reproducible. Furthermore, no "gold standard" exists with which a given impact can be compared to test its validity. Therefore questioning the entire threshold approach is not unreasonable. After all, some practitioners might say, with so much riding on the decision, could a simple whim or preference change everything? Skeptics note the capricious quality of human opinions and values and suggest that to depend on such a seemingly fleeting parameter is far too unreliable in the making of major medical decisions.

Those who trust the threshold approach concede that impact (or utility) is indeed subjective and in fact believe that this fact is exactly as it should be. After all, they reason, human values and feelings *should* guide the patient's choice, albeit in a scientifically accurate context. In fact the context of a mathematically sound construct clearly separates the facts from the feelings; failure to do so leaves behind a cold, "by-the-numbers" approach. If any individual must decide which of two health states is "worse," who better to do so than the patient, who stands to bear the consequences of the decision?

The bulk of available evidence and opinion supports the latter perspective. For example, Giesler and colleagues[7] compared a standard gamble approach with time trade-off, a linear placement-like technique, and another method called *willingness to pay* in 57 patients with advanced prostate cancer. They applied a mathematic model to determine the patients' consistency in rating certain health states considered internally equivalent based on previous responses. Although the researchers detected a substantial lack of precision in patient utility assignments (different patients possibly assigning different scores to the same outcome), most techniques performed consistently, sometimes approaching 90%. Other research has reported variation in utility scores, depending on which method was used to elicit them, but even these reports have noted a substantial consistency within any one method.[28]

An additional fact that may mitigate the inconsistencies among different methods is that the *absolute* value is not all that important in medical decision making. The impact for a harmful outcome is weighed against the impact for a beneficial outcome (harm versus improvement); only the *relative* score or *ratio* of the two scores matters. Thus a patient who is inclined to assign unexpectedly high or low scores to a side effect may be inclined equally dramatically toward the impact of an improvement. A certain balance emerges for a given patient in the application of this tool. In addition, use of one impact assessment tool per scenario makes sense, rather than use of a linear placement for the harm impact and a standard gamble for the improvement impact.

Thus threshold decision making is imperfect, but it is far superior to decision making based on "hunches" or pure intuition. At the very least the threshold method ensures that for all the vagaries of patient values and preferences, they are applied with a model that correctly accounts for evidence-based probabilities and proportionate comparison of risks and benefits.

## Dealing with Personal Value Systems

Most practitioners strive to avoid imposing on patients their own opinions about the impact of various outcomes. However, a practitioner's sharing of opinions in a nonauthoritarian context may be valuable. If a patient appears to assign an unexpectedly high or low impact to one of the outcomes under discussion, the practitioner's gentle verification that the patient understands the issues clearly and that their personal reasoning about the judgment is plausible is useful and even commendable.

Quill and Brody[22] note the following in a thoughtful article on patient autonomy:

> [By] taking the risk of informing patients about . . . [the physician's] own feelings, values, and recommendations, physicians can deepen and enrich medical decisions . . . Final choices belong to patients, but these choices gain meaning, richness, and accuracy if they are the result of a process of mutual influence and understanding between physician and patient.

Those practitioners who *obscure* patient values with their own do so at the risk of giving poor advice and compromising the quality of care. Those who blindly accept raw quantitative assessments of patient values also may provide less than optimal guidance. A practitioner's ideal approach may be to elicit explicitly patient values, using gentle and neutral coaxing and guidance, along with respectful concern. In addition, the practitioner may share personal experiences and judgment selectively. In any case, development of a useful threshold is necessary; this threshold may not be a perfect representation, but it certainly pays homage to the patient's world view and provides the best evidence available.

## SUMMARY

This chapter's discussion has focused on the type of evidence that is both the most common and the most complex encountered in medical practice. If readers are new to the concepts presented, a second reading may be useful. The discussion's essence boils down to the following facts:

1. Questions of therapy are framed to seek evidence about the improvements it causes, as well as side effects.
2. Therapy evidence can be retrieved efficiently, ideally from RCTs. It generally reflects the likelihood of the reduction of a bad outcome or the causation of side effects.
3. The applicability and validity of such evidence can be appraised efficiently.
4. The AT for any treatment and disease can be calculated as the best single parameter of its value. Estimating a patient's feelings about various related outcomes is an integral part of such a calculation.

## REFERENCES

1. Chan R, Hemeryck L, O'Regan M, and others: Oral versus intravenous antibiotics for community acquired lower respiratory tract infection in a general hospital: open, randomised controlled trial, *BMJ* 310:1360-1362, 1995.
2. Chiara S, Nobile MT, Vincenti M, and others: Advanced colorectal cancer in the elderly: results of consecutive trials with 5-fluorouracil-based chemotherapy, *Cancer Chemother Pharmacol* 42(4):336-340, 1998.
3. Downs JR and others: Primary prevention of acute coronary events with lovastatin in men and women with average cholesterol levels: results of AFCAPS/TexCAPS (Air Force/Texas Coronary Atherosclerosis Prevention Study), *JAMA* 279:1615-1622, 1998.
4. Fisher B and others: Tamoxifen for prevention of breast cancer: report of the national surgical adjuvant breast and bowel project p-1 study, *J Natl Cancer Inst* 90(18):1371-1388, 1998.
5. Fletcher RH, Fletcher SW, Wagner EH: *Clinical epidemiology—the essentials,* Baltimore, 1996, Williams & Wilkins.
6. Garg R, Yusuf S (for the Collaborative Group on ACE Inhibitor Trials): Overview of randomized trials of angiotensin-converting enzyme inhibitors on mortality and morbidity in patients with heart failure, *JAMA* 273:1450-1456, 1995.
7. Giesler RB and others: Assessing the performance of utility techniques in the absence of a gold standard, *Med Care* 37(6):580-588, 1999.
8. Gorelick PB and others: Prevention of a first stroke: a review of guidelines and a multidisciplinary consensus statement from the National Stroke Association, *JAMA* 281:1112-1120, 1999.
9. Haynes RB: Drug dependence in a journal club, *ACP J Club* A13-A15, 1999 (editorial).
10. Haynes RB and others: Developing optimal search strategies for detecting clinically sound studies in MEDLINE, *J Am Med Inform Assoc* 1(6):447-458, 1994.

11. Hardcastle JD and others: Randomised controlled trial of faecal-occult-blood screening for colorectal cancer, *Lancet* 348:1472-1477, 1996.

12. Hébert PC and others: A multicenter, randomized controlled clinical trial of transfusion requirements in critical care, *N Engl J Med* 340:409-417, 1999.

13. Kaiser L, Lew D, Hirschel B, and others: Effects of antibiotic treatment in the subset of common-cold patients who have bacteria in nasopharyngeal secretions, *Lancet* 347:1507-1510, 1996.

14. Knapp MJ and others: A 20-week randomized controlled trial of high-dose tacrine in patients with Alzheimer's disease, *JAMA* 271:985-991, 1994.

15. Kostis JB and others: Adverse effects of enalapril in the studies of left ventricular dysfunction (SOLVD), *Am Heart J* 131(2):350-355, 1996.

16. Executive Committee for the Asymptomatic Carotid Atherosclerosis (ACAS) Study: Endarterectomy for asymptomatic carotid artery stenosis, *JAMA* 273:1421-1428, 1995.

17. MERIT-HF Study Group: Effect of metoprolol CR/XL in chronic heart failure: metoprolol CR/XL randomised intervention trial in congestive Heart Failure (MERIT-HF), *Lancet* 353:2001-2007, 1999.

18. Bowers S and others: Ampicillin. In Hutchison and others (eds): *DRUGDEX© System,* Englewood, Colo, MICROMEDEX Inc (edition expires December 2000).

19. Mohammad JA and others: Ultrasound in the diagnosis and management of fluid collection complications following abdominoplasty, *Ann Plast Surg* 41:498-502, 1998.

20. Moher D, Jones A, Cook DJ, and others: Does quality of reports of randomised trials affect estimates of intervention efficacy reported in meta-analyses? *Lancet* 352:609-613, 1998.

21. Pauker SC, Kassirer JP: The threshold approach to clinical decision making, *N Engl J Med* 302:1109-1117, 1980.

22. Quill TE, Brody H: Physician recommendations and patient autonomy: finding a balance between physician power and patient choice, *Ann Intern Med* 125:763-769, 1996.

23. Rogers SL, Doody RS, Mohs RC, and others: Donepezil improves cognition and global function in Alzheimer disease: a 15-week, double-blind, placebo-controlled study (Donepezil Study Group), *Arch Intern Med* 158(9):1021-1031, 1998.

24. Sackett DL and others: Evidence based medicine: what it is and what it isn't, *BMJ* 312:71-72, 1996.

25. Sackett DL and others: *Evidence-based medicine: how to practice and teach EBM,* ed 2, New York, 2000, Churchill Livingstone.

26. Schulz KF, Chalmers I, Hayes RJ, and others: Empirical evidence of bias: dimensions of methodologic quality associated with estimates of treatment effects in controlled trials, *JAMA* 273:408-412, 1995.

27. Schulz KF: Assessing allocation concealment and blinding in randomized controlled trials: why bother? *ACP J Club* 132(2):A11-A12, 2000.

28. Stiggelbout AM and others: Utility assessment in cancer patients: adjustment of time tradeoff scores for the utility of life years and comparison with standard gamble scores, *Med Decis Making* 14(1):82-90, 1994.

29. Yoshida H and others: Interferon therapy reduces the risk for hepatocellular carcinoma: national surveillance program of cirrhotic and noncirrhotic patients with chronic hepatitis C in Japan, *Ann Intern Med* 131:174-181, 1999.

30. Zeneca pharmaceuticals (advertisement), *Ann Intern Med* 129:(inside cover), 1998.

## RECOMMENDED READINGS

Blogg MW: *Bibliography of the writings of Sir William Osler,* Baltimore, 1921, The Cord Baltimore Press.

Boston Area Anticoagulation Trial for Atrial Fibrillation Investigators: The effect of low-dose warfarin on the risk of stroke in patients with nonrheumatic atrial fibrillation, *N Engl J Med* 323:1505-1511, 1990.

Chrysant SG, Fagan T, Glazer R, and others: Effects of benazepril and hydrochlorothiazide, given alone and in low- and high-dose combinations, on blood pressure in patients with hypertension, *Arch Fam Med* 5(1):17-24 [discussion 25], 1996.

Gage BF, Cardinalli AB, Albers GW, and others: Cost-effectiveness of warfarin and aspirin for prophylaxis of stroke in patients with nonvalvular atrial fibrillation, *JAMA* 274:1839-1845, 1995.

Goldberg AI, Dunlay MC, Sweet CS: Safety and tolerability of losartan potassium, an angiotensin II receptor antagonist, compared with hydrochlorothiazide, atenolol, felodipine ER, and angiotensin-converting enzyme inhibitors for the treatment of systemic hypertension, *Am J Cardiol* 75(12):793-795, 1995.

Gross RA: *Making medical decisions,* Philadelphia, 1999, American College of Physicians.

Mazur DJ, Hickam DH: Patients' preferences for risk disclosure and role in decision making for invasive medical procedures, *J Gen Intern Med* 12(2):114-117, 1997.

Sox HC and others: *Medical decision making,* Stoneham, Mass, 1998, Butterworth-Heineman.

# CHAPTER 4

# *Diagnostic Testing*

## INTRODUCTION

Traditionally, medical professionals have conceptualized diagnostic testing as a means to make a diagnosis. To the extent that the phrase *make a diagnosis* implies certainty, this perspective may not be accurate. For evidence-based decision making (EDBM) a preferable concept is that of "confident uncertainty." This chapter focuses on *confidence* in decisions in the face of *uncertainty* about the diagnosis.

A suitable working explanation for why practitioners perform tests can be summarized in the following statement:

Testing is performed to improve the estimate of the likelihood of a diagnosis, compared with the estimate of its likelihood before the test is performed.

Another important point this discussion aims to define is how diagnostic testing interacts with the action threshold (AT; see Chapter 3) to form the final link in a decision analysis. A practitioner's decision about whether to proceed with a test and how to apply its results both are linked intimately to the AT.

# *Components of Diagnostic Test Decisions*

## PRELIMINARY CONCEPTS

### Gold Standard

Every diagnosis must have a gold standard, or a series of findings or criteria on which the diagnosis rests. Sometimes this standard is obvious—a biopsy result, culture, or unique set of clinical findings. In other cases (for example, fibromyalgia or chronic fatigue syndrome) the criteria are complex and controversial and often consist of sets of symptoms and findings hardly unique to that disease. For this discussion the gold standard refers to those findings that define the presence of a disease with as much certainty as is currently available.

**Prevalence**  The prevalence of a disease, usually expressed as probability, is its likelihood in a given population at a specific *point* in time according to the gold standard. In the case of chronic diseases this concept may include individuals who developed the disease long ago, along with those who developed it the previous day.

**Incidence**  The incidence of a disease, usually expressed as probability, is the percentage of patients newly diagnosed with the disease according to the gold standard within a defined *period* of time. In the case of chronic diseases, only those patients *newly diagnosed* within the time period are included. In the case of self-limited diseases, only those whose diagnoses are made within the time period are included.

### Understanding the Numeric Parameters of Diagnostic Testing

**Pretest Likelihood**  A critical element in the understanding of diagnostic testing relates to the practitioner's estimate of the likelihood of a diagnosis *before* testing, known as the *pretest likelihood*. With the exception of "perfect" diagnostic tests (that is, those that are never wrong), all diagnostic tests operate on the pretest likelihood. Regardless of whether a test alters the pretest estimate greatly or slightly, upward or downward, the substrate on which tests operate is always the same—the pretest likelihood estimate. In essence it is the individual's "index of suspicion."

Typically the pretest likelihood is expressed simply as the percentage of all patients with similar findings who on final diagnosis actually have the disease in question. As with all likelihood, the number also may be expressed as odds. (This concept will be discussed in greater detail in later sections of this chapter.)

**Normal, Abnormal, Positive, Negative**  A test is said to be positive when its result does not fall within a specified range of "normal" values. The values in question may be defined by the range within which 95% of individuals without the disease fall (according to the gold standard). As with confidence intervals (see Chapter 1) the 95% figure is arbitrary but customary.

In the case of a gold-standard test (the one defining the disease in question), ideally all individuals with the disease fall outside the normal range and all individuals without the disease fall within the normal range. Practically, gold standards for many diseases are a bit tarnished, and occasional errors in their predictions can come to light only at autopsy or under other extreme circumstances; gold standards are the best available measures but are not always perfect.

Many tests are reported in a scalar manner; that is, rather than as a simple positive or negative, they are reported numerically along a scale. The classic example is that of hematocrit, the percent of volume of a blood sample that is composed of red blood cells. Normal values may be in the range of 36% to 48%. When the value reflects a biologic phenomenon, reason dictates that values outside the range by a very small amount may not have the same strength in predicting a disease (such as iron deficiency) as values far outside the normal range. Similarly, values just barely within the normal range may not provide as much reassurance about the absence of disease as values squarely within the midrange of normal.

**Sensitivity**  Sensitivity is the percent of all individuals with the disease who have abnormal test results; mnemonics include how often the test is positive in disease (PID) and abnormal if diseased (AID).

When a test is less than 100% sensitive, some individuals with the disease have normal test results; they will be "missed" by the test. These are known as the *false negatives;* they look healthy according to the test, but the test is wrong. Their numbers are calculated with the following formula:

$$1 - \text{Sensitivity}$$

Importantly, the definition of sensitivity says nothing about how often the test is abnormal in individuals *without* the disease. A positive result is a *false positive* if it occurs in a *healthy* individual (see following discussion). Thus by itself, sensitivity is insufficient for describing how powerful a test might be.

**Specificity**  Specificity reflects how likely a test result is to be normal in healthy individuals (without the disease in question). The standard mnemonic refers to how often the test is normal in health (NIH).

When a test is negative in health (as it should be) less than 100% of the time, some healthy individuals have abnormal test results, described by the following equation:

$$1 - \text{Specificity}$$

This important group of healthy individuals is composed of the false positives. They "appear" diseased according to the test results, but the results are wrong in their cases.

A highly specific test may be normal in healthy individuals almost all the time; unfortunately, it may also be normal in *diseased* patients far too often. Thus by itself, specificity is insufficient in the assessment of how powerful a test is.

*Limitations of sensitivity and specificity*   A highly sensitive test is best at ruling *out* a disease when the result is negative. Conversely, the ability of a test to rule a disease *in* cannot be judged by its sensitivity; although the test is abnormal in almost all individuals *with* disease, it also may pick up many people *without* the disease. Unfortunately, practitioners cannot always expect sensitive tests to be negative and specific tests to be positive.

> ### Example
>
> A positive strep culture is found in 95% of individuals with acute strep throat. Thus if a strep culture is negative, the presence of acute strep throat is highly unlikely. Approximately 15% of adults harbor streptococci in their throat as part of their normal bacteria, with no disease present. Thus up to 15% of the individuals who test positive may not even have strep throat but rather may be mere "carriers."

The acronym *SnNout* can help readers remember this concept. (**Sen**sitive tests when **N**egative rule disease ***out.***) Practitioners rule out (SnNout) a disease by performing a highly sensitive test that returns a normal result.

A highly specific test is best at ruling a disease *in* when the result is positive. Conversely, the ability of a test to rule a disease *out* cannot be judged by its specificity; although almost all individuals with abnormal results actually have the disease, many others with the disease may provide normal results.

> ### Example
>
> Almost all individuals with a combination of acute pleuritic chest pain, shortness of breath, normal chest x-ray, and high-probability lung scan have a pulmonary embolus; this combination of findings is highly specific for this disease. However, many individuals with pulmonary embolus lack one or more of these findings, so if you rely on the combination present to make your diagnosis, you will miss many cases.

The acronym *SpPin* can help readers remember this concept (**Sp**ecific tests when **P**ositive rule disease ***in***).

Many practitioners (myself included) find remembering how and when to apply sensitivity and specificity confusing, not to mention determining how to combine both concepts into a practical decision tool. A much better way to consider the terms is to merge them into a single parameter, the *likelihood ratio (LR)*. (This concept will be discussed fully in the decision-making section of this chapter.) Sensitivity and specificity should be considered the raw evidence to seek for diagnostic tests. However, practitioners should recognize that they are used best to calculate LRs, not as stand-alone tools.

## Pretest Estimation Data from Diagnostic Test Studies— A Free Lunch?

Lying within most studies of diagnostic tests is a nugget often overlooked—the percent of all individuals who have abnormal gold-standard test results, which provides an excellent approximation of the pretest likelihood of the disease in question. Practitioners may use this figure as a starting point for their own estimates for the individual patient; to the extent that the patient is well represented in the study population, the practitioner's work in this regard largely is completed. As discussed in the decision section, the number may need a bit of modification, but at least this percentage puts the practitioner in the right ballpark.

Many new students of EBDM become skeptical when faced with the importance of pretest estimates because they perceive the estimates as little more than pure guesswork. However, guessing is not the case if the practitioner knows where to look—in the evidence about the test. One might consider using the prevalence of the disease in the general population to estimate pretest likelihood. This use is misleading because a physician is unlikely to "work up" a disease in a patient who has the same risk of the disease as does the general population; indeed something made that physician suspect the presence of the disease, so the estimate almost always is higher than the general disease prevalence. Good evidence about tests examines a population *likely to be tested in real life* (that is, with a suspicion of disease similar to the physician's suspicion).

Fortunately, another source of pretest estimates also often is available—evidence about differential diagnosis. Such studies take typical populations of individuals with a particular symptom or syndrome, apply all appropriate diagnostic tests to all individuals, and then report the percentage of the group with each of the various diagnoses that comprises the usual differential diagnosis list (that is, those other diseases the practitioner might also consider in appraising patients with similar presentations).

In summary, the evidence readers must seek to evaluate diagnostic tests includes sensitivity and specificity (to calculate LRs), as well as pretest likelihood. The next section examines the manner in which studies of diagnostic tests are designed.

# *Evidence about Diagnostic Tests*

## UNDERSTANDING CLINICAL STUDIES ABOUT DIAGNOSTIC TESTS

Diagnostic tests generally are studied through use of a cohort study design. The steps are as follows:

- Identify a group (cohort) of individuals that typifies the population in which the test would be applied in a clinical setting. Establish in advance the parameters that constitute a normal and abnormal result whenever practical. Ensure that the participants have not yet received the gold-standard test when they enter the study; those who have already undergone the gold-standard test usually are not highly representative of the "typical population" group, the target group for the experimental test.
- Apply both the experimental test and the gold-standard test to all cohort participants. Results of this test generate two subcohorts—those individuals with normal results (no disease) and those with abnormal results (disease). The situation is illustrated in Figure 4.1. Traditionally this distribution is illustrated in a table with two rows and two columns (the "2 × 2" table), as shown in Figure 4.2. Box A shows all individuals with the disease

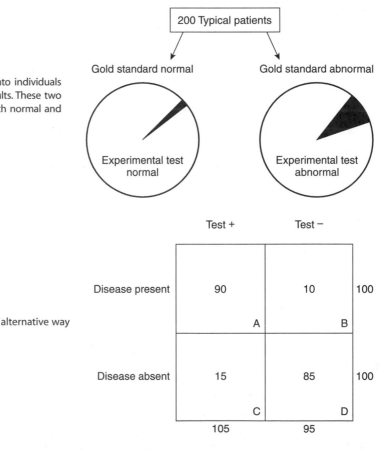

**Figure 4.1** The study group is subdivided into individuals with normal and abnormal gold-standard results. These two groups in turn are divided into individuals with normal and abnormal experimental-test results.

**Figure 4.2** The standard "2 × 2" table is an alternative way to portray the results shown in Figure 4.1.

|  | Test + | Test − |  |
|---|---|---|---|
| Disease present | 90 (A) | 10 (B) | 100 |
| Disease absent | 15 (C) | 85 (D) | 100 |
|  | 105 | 95 |  |

whose test results are positive, whereas box D illustrates those without disease whose test results are negative.

- Maintain blinding as to the clinical features and test results for both participants and researchers whenever possible. If interpretation of the test results involves a subjective component, blinding is an absolute criterion.
- Analyze the results to determine the percentage of participants with abnormal gold-standard results (those with disease) who also demonstrated abnormal experimental results (sensitivity), as well as the percentage of individuals with normal gold-standard results (those without disease) who also had normal experimental results (specificity).

Other important considerations for the study's designers are to ensure that the individuals with normal gold-standard results are similar to those with abnormal gold-standard results other than in respect to the disease in question.

## RETRIEVING EVIDENCE ABOUT DIAGNOSTIC TESTS

### The Master Evidence Question

The Master Evidence Question for diagnostic test evidence is as follows:

*In individuals representative of mine, what are the sensitivity and specificity values of this test for this disease?*

### Search Strategies

The evidence may exist as sensitivity and specificity or as LRs, all of which are described in this section. As always the user should begin the search with a preappraised resource, such as Best Evidence or a similar database. The Cochrane Library, so useful for treatments, is not useful for diagnostic test evidence. If this initial database search fails to retrieve sufficient relevant evidence, or as a check for further evidence, the user should consult MEDLINE.

The two-pass approach in the search for evidence in MEDLINE was discussed in Chapter 3, and the same principles work well for diagnostic test evidence. The user begins with a broad search to capture almost all articles of interest and then filter them down to a usable number. Following is the suggested search syntax:

**Pass 1:** Keywords AND diagnos* OR sens*
**Pass 2:** Previous search AND sensitivity AND specificity

NOTE: Depending on the context, addition of the phrase *OR differential diagnosis* to both passes may prove useful. As noted previously, this addition is important when the physician requires help with the pretest estimate.

Following is a review of an example that illustrates not only the use of the correct syntax but also some pitfalls users should avoid. To find evidence (sensitivity and specificity for calculation of LRs) about the antigliadin antibody test for a diagnosis of sprue (a disease leading to digestive malabsorption) the following search strategy seems reasonable:

**Pass 1:** antigliadin AND sprue AND diagnos* OR sens*
*Results:* 2466, many of which are entirely irrelevant, including one on synthesized tinnitus

What went wrong? Note the absence of parentheses in the search query. The search engine interpreted the search as follows: find every article with the words *antigliadin* and *sprue* and *diagnos** or any article containing *sens**. In other words, any article with the words *sensitivity, sensation, sensational,* and other similar words was included. Rephrasing the search criteria with parentheses makes it unambiguous:

antigliadin AND sprue AND (diagnos* OR sens*)

This query turns up 75 articles. A brief scan shows most of them to be relevant.

The diagnosis *sprue* also goes by the names *gluten enteropathy, celiac disease,* and *coeliac disease,* to name a few. Because the previous query did *not* use a wild-card notation (for example, *sprue**), the search engine checked the term against the medical subject heading (MeSH) index in the MEDLINE phrase list and thus did the cross-referencing automatically (see Chapter 3). Adding the wild card would have suppressed this cross-referencing. Following is the same search but with phrase and MeSH referencing suppressed by virtue of the wild-card addition:

**Pass 1:** antigliadin AND sprue* AND (diagnos* OR sens*)
*Results:* 2 articles; 73 of the 75 relevant articles are missed, a point to keep in mind.

Now pass 2 is applied to the 75 previously cited articles. Clicking on the *history* link in the PubMed page notifies the user that the previous search was assigned the number 3. So the second search reads as follows:

**Pass 2:** #3 AND sensitivity AND specificity
*Results:* 34 articles, a number easily scanned in a few minutes; among these articles are several that appear to be quite appropriate.*

Consider another example of the two-pass searching method.

| *Example* |

You wonder whether a normal sedimentation rate is sufficient to rule out temporal arteritis in a patient who has highly suggestive symptoms.

---

*An interesting aside is that one article[8] used a cohort whose members were proven (via biopsy and the blood test) to have the disease. The study's authors then presented predictive values for the group. Predictive values are applicable only to a group with the same disease prevalence as the study group, so these figures are only usable by a physician who knows the patient in question has the disease. The illogical design of such a study underscores the importance of careful appraisal of the evidence before it is applied.

Thus you are especially interested in SnNout—high sensitivity to rule out the condition with a negative result.

**Pass 1:** temporal arteritis AND sedimentation rate AND (diagnos* OR sens*)
*Results:* 167

Note the lack of wild-card characters for terms that might match to a phrase or synonym that you mean to include (that is, phrase and MeSH matching being active).

**Pass 2:** #1 AND diagnosis AND sensitivity
*Results:* 12; after scanning them, you find this list to be highly relevant, and one even provides a mathematic model for predicting a negative biopsy.[2] (It indirectly addresses the present question by finding a normal sedimentation rate insufficient to rule out the diagnosis.) Other articles show very poor sensitivity for this test.

You conclude that the sedimentation rate has a low sensitivity and thus does not rule out the diagnosis in this suspicious presentation.

The reader is encouraged to practice with imaginary case scenarios. Students of EBDM should be creative in the use of the key search terms for a topic but try to keep the strategy terms (that is, *diagnos\**, *sens\**, *sensitivity*, and *specificity*) constant.

In addition, readers are urged to examine studies with cohorts resembling that of the patient in question and then review the disease prevalence in that group to get a sense of the pretest likelihood estimates. For example, in the temporal arteritis scenario, one study examined all patients referred for biopsy at a major referral center.[5] The reader can presume these individuals to be a high pretest likelihood group, and indeed the patients had a prevalence of 26% for probable disease on biopsy. The reader may use this percentage as the high end for the pretest estimate, modified for the specifics of the case at hand.

## JUDGING THE SUITABILITY OF DIAGNOSTIC TEST EVIDENCE

The applicability and validity of diagnostic test evidence should be assessed carefully before it is used to make decisions. The criteria in general usage in evidence-based medicine (EBM) circles are presented below, drawn largely from Jaeschke and colleagues.[3-4]

### Assessing Applicability

For diagnostic evidence the physician should ask a few pointed questions to assess a study's applicability.

#### Are the Patients Like My Patient?
*Do the patients in the study group resemble my patient demographically and biologically?*

Some tests are more accurate for certain age or gender categories than for others. For example, exercise stress testing is less specific in women than in men; sedimentation rates normally rise with age.

*Does the disease gamut studied include my patient's disease profile?*

Although this criterion is considered a validity issue in many discussions, it seems to be an applicability issue as well. That is, if the patient would not have met the criteria for entry into the study, the practitioner must decide on a comfort level in using the results.

The term *gamut* should be used to mean both the severity of disease and its duration. Early, late, mild, and advanced disease each may generate different sensitivities and specificities for the same test. The practitioner should ensure that all factors are assessed in relationship to the patient in question, when appropriate.

### Is the Test Realistic to Consider?

*Can the test be done comparably and practically in your locale?*

If a test is so esoteric or impractical (expensive, risky, painful) that it would not be advised regardless of its accuracy, the evidence is essentially inapplicable. Positron emission tomography (PET) scans are an example of this phenomenon in most locations. PET scans describe a powerful but largely experimental imaging technique; they may be quite useful for selected patients, but they are so uncommonly available as to be impractical.

## Assessing Validity

Under the assumption that the practitioner judged the evidence to be applicable, that evidence should be appraised as to whether it actually measures what it claims to measure.

### Was the Test Measured Blindly against a Biologically Independent and Uniformly Applied Gold Standard?

Practitioners should ensure that the individuals in the study group who are assumed to have the disease in question are identified with the gold-standard test. In fact, *every* subject should receive the same gold-standard test, regardless of the results of the study test. If the gold-standard test is performed only on a subset of all subjects (for example, only those whose experimental test results were abnormal), the false negatives for the population at large will be missed.

| *Example* |

A study on treadmill testing for coronary disease was performed. Each participant whose treadmill test was abnormal received coronary catheterization. The test was reported to be highly sensitive but only moderately specific.

What of those who had coronary disease but whose treadmill tests were normal? Some of these individuals may have had coronary disease that would have been detected on catheterization. With this faulty methodology the practitioner has no way of knowing the percentage of subjects with disease who were missed by the test (false-negative rate).

Blinding is an especially important criterion if the interpretation of either test (the study test or the gold standard) has any subjective aspects; the researchers should be blind to the results of the study test when interpreting the gold-standard test and blind to the gold-standard results when interpreting the study test results.

Readers are reminded that the concept known as *interobserver variability* was discussed in Chapter 3. This variability can arise as a validity problem when the interpretation of a test result has a subjective component. The measure of this variability (the agreement observed above that which is expected by chance alone) is the kappa ($\kappa-$) value, 0.6 being a decent value and 0.8 or higher being excellent.

*Is the gold standard a different procedure biologically from the study test?*

If each test is simply a different way to describe the same finding, the tests' correlation might reflect their similarity only. For example, the practitioner who wanted to assess a test for the presence of anemia could define the gold-standard test as the hematocrit. The study test might be a hemoglobin level. However, for most anemias the hemoglobin simply reflects the hematocrit level and vice versa; they both respond to iron levels and other similar factors. Thus the finding of a very high sensitivity and specificity for hemoglobin would reflect less that it is a good test for anemia than it does that the test in many ways is a variation of the gold standard itself.

These questions constitute primary validity criteria; if the criteria are not met substantially, the validity of the study may be compromised.

## Was the Population in the Study Reflective of Patients for Whom I Would Probably Use this Test?

This question refers primarily to the setting from which the participants were drawn. Although this factor may be an applicability issue more than one of validity, primary-care providers should beware of evidence drawn from tertiary referral populations and vice versa. This evidence can lead to mathematically valid conclusions that can mislead the patient; the baseline population likely contains a very different profile of competing diagnoses.

At the other extreme, populations in which the practitioner has little or no reason to suspect the presence of a disease usually are not the best proving grounds for new tests (except for screening tests, which are discussed near the end of this chapter). Studying the test in populations with findings likely to lead to consideration of the test in question is a better idea. Thus an antinuclear cytoplasmic antibody test for Wegener's granulomatosis should not be assessed in a general population but rather in one under assessment for vasculitis and other suspicious presentations.

### Is the Testing Methodology Fully Disclosed?

For proprietary or technical reasons, certain diagnostic procedures may not be described sufficiently to allow others to reproduce the procedures. This issue should raise a red flag in the physician's mind for at least the following two reasons:

1. If no one else has the means to validate or even reproduce the findings, the physician must rely totally on the single source for evidence. If not generally a question of integrity, this situation certainly becomes a question of validity because of how often one group's results fail to confirm that of another group in scientific research.
2. Another reason to be cautious about incompletely revealed methodology is that subtle issues of technique, skill levels, and other technical elements may render a test impractical or unreliable except in certain hands. The physician and patient need to know of any such limitations before relying on evidence for a test that may be performed quite differently from the manner used in the original research.

Once a test is studied and its parameters established, verification of the results with a second, independent but comparable group of subjects provides reassurance. Finding similar results in the second population ensures the physician that the initial results can be generalized.

The appraisal process for diagnostic testing is summarized in Figure 4.3.

## UNDERSTANDING RESULTS OF DIAGNOSTIC TEST EVIDENCE—LIKELIHOOD RATIOS

### Why Bother with Likelihood Ratios?

Virtually all evidence pertaining to tests reports sensitivity and specificity. Unfortunately, these parameters are not sufficient or intuitive enough by themselves to determine the power of a test. For purposes of this discussion *power* reflects the ability of a test to alter the pretest estimate of the disease likelihood either upward (when the result is abnormal) or downward (when it is normal). Highly experienced statisticians can assess power from these numbers alone, but this process involves cumbersome calculations. Attempts to render test parameters more intuitive have included receiver operator curves, in which the true-positive rate is plotted against the false-positive rate. However, I have yet to meet a practitioner who finds such tools practical; see Sox[6] for a lucid discussion of this area, if desired. Clearly, a single, cohesive value that incorporates both sensitivity and specificity into a single parameter is needed, and the LR serves this purpose nicely.

### Likelihood Ratios Demystified

Two types of LR exist—positive and negative. Every test has both types, and the practitioner must use whichever one applies to the test result under consider-

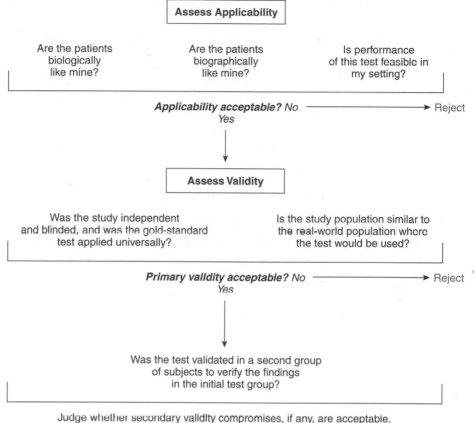

**Figure 4.3** Summary of appraisal of evidence on tests. Note that *accept* and *reject* are rarely absolute but rather reflect the extremes of how closely a finding approximates the "true" effect.

ation (that is, positive LR when the result is positive; negative LR when the result is negative).

*Positive likelihood ratio (LR+):* The clearest conceptual definition is that the LR+ is the probability that a positive is *right,* divided by the probability that it is *wrong.* In other words, it is the ratio of true positives to false positives.

$$LR+ = \frac{\text{sensitivity}}{(1 - \text{specificity})}$$

The LR+ is always greater than 1 for any rational test. It may be expressed as follows: "of all patients with a positive result, X are correct for every one that is incorrect," where X is the LR+.

*Negative likelihood ratio (LR−):* Conversely, the LR− is the probability that a negative test result is *wrong,* compared with the probability that the result is *right.* It is the proportion of false negatives to true negatives and is always less than 1 for any rational test.

$$LR- = \frac{(1 - \text{sensitivity})}{\text{specificity}}$$

The LR− is expressed as follows: "of all patients with a negative result, Y are incorrect for every one that is correct," where Y is the LR−.

The reader must know the sensitivity and specificity evidence to calculate LRs. Two of the few formulas readers are advised to memorize in this book are the previously stated LR equations (the others being the odds-to-probability conversions in Chapter 1, the AT formula in Chapter 3, and the posttest odds formula in the following discussion).

So what constitutes a good or bad LR? The answer, of course, is context sensitive. However, the reader may look reasonably at an LR+ of 4 or greater as somewhat valuable and values of 10 and above as quite good. An LR− of 0.6 or less is somewhat useful, whereas a value of 0.1 or below is quite good. Clearly, however situations exist in which lesser or greater values may prove perfectly satisfactory.

# *Helping the Patient Decide*

## USING DIAGNOSTIC TEST EVIDENCE IN MEDICAL DECISIONS

### The Master Decision Question

The Master Decision Question for diagnosis is as follows:

> *Given my pretest estimate of the likelihood of disease, could this test move that likelihood across the AT for the treatment I am considering?*

The implication of the master decision question is that if a test could change the physician's mind about whether to treat, it might benefit the patient. That is, if the physician were inclined initially to treat the patient but would decide against treatment if the results were normal, the test is valuable; similarly, if the physician would be inclined initially *not* to treat but would choose treatment if the test were abnormal, performance of the test is valuable in this situation as well.

The decision-making value of a test rests in its ability to refine the pretest likelihood of disease. After testing is performed, the estimate rises with a positive result and drops with a negative result. All that is needed is a decision target for which to aim; that target is the AT.

The AT is an approximation of a treatment's risks and benefits. The lower the AT, the better the overall outcomes from treatment. In regards to diagnosis the AT represents the likelihood of diagnosis above which treatment (as opposed to observation, for example) is the best decision and below which observation is the best decision. Use of the word *best* in the aforementioned definition refers to that decision most likely to lead to the patient's preferred outcomes, on average.

This concept (the AT) enables the practitioner to provide patients with beneficial advice. It shuns any attempt to predict outcomes with certainty but provides great certainty in the correctness of the decision. Individuals deal with such apparent paradoxes routinely in other aspects of life. For example, a poker player with a very high hand (such as a straight flush) likely would bet a considerable sum on that hand. The player *knows* that this bet usually is the best thing to do to win the game. The player does not know whether the hand will prove to be a winner (although it is judged as highly likely), but the player is certain that betting is wise.

The physician also has certainty that betting on the treatment is the right decision despite uncertainty about the outcome. Given the AT and the pretest likelihood, the situation can be portrayed graphically as shown in Figure 4.4.

In this figure the pretest likelihood is lower than the AT. With testing, as shown by the "spread line," a positive test result would raise the disease likelihood to a level higher than the AT. Thus before testing is performed, the physician would be inclined not to treat, whereas that physician is more likely to choose treatment after performing the test. If the pretest likelihood had been *higher* than the AT and if a negative test would have dropped the likelihood *below* the AT, the converse interpretation would apply; thus before testing was performed, the physician likely would have chosen treatment, whereas after testing occurred, the decision to observe the patient only would be more likely.

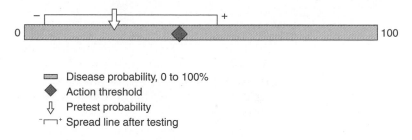

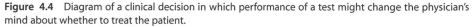

Figure 4.4 Diagram of a clinical decision in which performance of a test might change the physician's mind about whether to treat the patient.

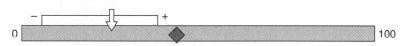

**Figure 4.5** Diagram of a clinical decision in which performance of a test would *not* change the physician's mind about whether to treat the patient.

A corollary of the situation presented in Figure 4.4 is that if a test might change the physician's mind, it is worth doing. Then if a test would *not* change the physician's mind, should it *not* be performed? Consider the situation illustrated in Figure 4.5.

This situation begins similarly to that presented in Figure 4.4. Before testing is performed, the physician would not choose treatment over nontreatment because the pretest likelihood is less than the AT. After testing is done, the disease likelihood increases if the result is positive, but only to a point *that remains below the AT.* Thus after testing is performed, the physician still would not choose the treatment for the patient. Why do the test?

Indeed the physician probably should *not* perform the test because it has no decision value. Yet day after day, physicians do the exact opposite. If these actions are due to incomplete understanding of the principles involved in decision making, the time, money, and resources simply are wasted. A solid understanding of these principles can result in a more efficient, accurate, and consistent approach to clinical medicine.

Sometimes the physician may elect legitimately to perform a test despite a decision analysis suggesting the test is of no value. One reason for this action is the so-called value of knowing. Even if treatment choices would not be affected by performance of the test, results can provide prognostic information, reassurance for the patient that cannot be provided in the absence of the results, and other interpersonal issues too numerous to list. More often, however, my experience has found that such explanations are unconvincing; a better approach is for the physician to communicate to the patient the reasons why the test is not a good option. Again in my experience, patients are surprisingly receptive to such explanations.

> ### Example
>
> Your patient has requested a throat culture to determine the presence of strep throat, a test you believe is unwise. You tell her the following: "Mrs. Jones, your request for a throat culture is very reasonable. However, a strep culture is not a perfect test; it misses some cases and provides false-positive results in others, and treatment can have side effects. Based on my exam and your overall situation, even with a positive culture, your likelihood of having strep throat still would be so low that the risks of treatment would outweigh its benefits. I suggest that you wait a few days, take some acetaminophen for discomfort, and get back to me if things are not going well. That way, we can avoid the potential side effects of an antibiotic with very little risk of the disease worsening."

To summarize this discussion the physician should decide on a course of action based on the pretest estimate (that is, determination of whether that estimate is above or below the AT). Next, using the tools discussed in the following section, the physician should decide whether applying the test has the potential to move the patient across the AT (from above it to below or *vice versa*). If the test does carry this potential, it is worth performing; if not, the test is not worth doing.

The next section focuses on the means by which the physician can apply the actual evidence to decision making with confidence. Following the discussion are several examples by which the reader can learn to perform this simple process mentally.

### Predicting the Posttest Likelihood with Likelihood Ratios

For purposes of calculation this discussion focuses on likelihood in terms of odds, not probability. (Readers may consult Chapter 1 for a review of odds skills.)

The main conversion formulas for odds versus probability are as follows:

$$\text{Odds} = \frac{\text{probability}}{(1 - \text{probability})}$$

and

$$\text{Probability} = \frac{\text{odds}}{(1 + \text{odds})}$$

In addition, probability uses a 0-to-1 scale. Odds are chances *for* something divided by chances *against* them, whereas probability describes chances *for* something divided by *all* chances. A key point in this discussion is the following formula (which readers are advised to memorize):

$$\text{Posttest odds} = \text{pretest odds} \times \text{LR}$$

This simple formula is actually all an individual needs to understand the impact of diagnostic tests. Together with the AT concept, it provides the basic tools of most bedside decision analysis.

Some readers may recall the concept of predictive value when reviewing the previous formula. Predictive value (positive or negative) is an alternative used to calculate the likelihood of a disease with given a test result. At least the following two reasons exist why use of the odds approach instead of predictive values is encouraged:

1. The formula for predictive values is cumbersome, remembered by few, and all but impossible to perform mentally, as follows:

$$\text{Positive predictive value} = \frac{(\text{sensitivity} \times \text{pretest probability})}{(\text{sensitivity} \times \text{pretest probability}) + (1 - \text{specificity}) \times (1 - \text{pretest probability})}$$

2. Predictive values reported in the medical literature are tied to a single, fixed pretest probability. Not often does a patient have the same pretest likelihood as the value used in the initial study. LRs, on the other hand, can be applied to *any* pretest odds. Thus a practitioner who is provided a predictive value for a particular test from the literature should not use that value before confirming that the presumed pretest likelihood is the same as that of the patient in question.

### Practicing the Calculation of Posttest Odds

Because of its importance in decision analysis, the ability to use LRs to predict the likelihood of disease after a test result is known warrants emphasis. Table 4.1

## TABLE 4.1
### Probability/Odds Practice Problems

| Pretest Probability | Pretest Odds | Test Sensitivity | Test Specificity | LR+ | LR− | Posttest Probability | |
|---|---|---|---|---|---|---|---|
| | | | | | | Positive | Negative |
| 0.25 | | 0.9 | 0.85 | | | | |
| 0.8 | | 0.9 | 0.85 | | | | |
| 0.33 | | 0.9 | 0.7 | | | | |
| 0.5 | | 0.75 | 0.75 | | | | |
| 0.1 | | 0.95 | 0.95 | | | | |
| 0.02 | | 0.8 | 0.6 | | | | |
| 0.1 | | 0.85 | 0.5 | | | | |

*LR,* Likelihood ratio, *LR+,* positive likelihood ratio, *LR−,* negative likelihood ratio.
Calculating the missing values is a four-step process, as follows:

1. Convert pretest probability to pretest odds using the *probability ÷ (1 − probability)* equation.
2. Calculate LR+ using the equation *sensitivity ÷ (1 − specificity)* and the LR − using the equation *(1 − sensitivity) ÷ specificity.*
3. Calculate posttest odds with the equation *pretest odds × LR.*
4. Convert back to probability using the *odds ÷ (1 + odds)* equation.

features a series of practice cases to familiarize readers with this technique. The correct responses are provided in Table 4.2, but readers will benefit most by working through the problems before consulting the answers. Rounding off is acceptable, and probabilities always should be converted to a 0-to-1 scale.

Because pretest likelihood generally is accepted as probability, the practice problems begin with that assumption. The goal is to calculate the probability of disease after the test is performed, both for positive and negative results. The trick to this calculation without a resort to the predictive values is to convert to odds before the calculation is performed, as follows:

- Convert pretest probability to pretest odds using the following formula:

$$\frac{Probability}{(1 - Probability)}$$

*Example:* Probability of 0.4 converts to 0.4 ÷ (1 − 0.4) = 0 .67 (odds).
- Calculate LR+ and LR− using the following respective formulas:

$$\frac{Sensitivity}{(1 - Specificity)}$$

$$\frac{(1 - Sensitivity)}{Specificity}$$

*Example:* If sensitivity is 0.8 and specificity is 0.6, then LR+ is 0.8 ÷ (1 − 0.6), or 2; LR− is (1 − 0.8) ÷ 0.6, or 0.33.
- Calculate posttest odds using the following formula:

$$Pretest\ odds \times LR$$

*Example:* Using the previous values, posttest odds when the test is positive are 0.67 × 2, or 1.3. If the test is negative, use 0.67 × 0.33, or 0.2.

## TABLE 4.2
### Probability/Odds Practice Problem Solutions

| Pretest Probability | Pretest Odds | Test Sensitivity | Test Specificity | LR+ | LR− | Posttest Probability | |
|---|---|---|---|---|---|---|---|
| | | | | | | Positive | Negative |
| 0.25 | 0.33 | 0.9 | 0.85 | 6 | 0.12 | 0.66 | 0.038 |
| 0.8 | 4 | 0.9 | 0.85 | 6 | 0.12 | 0.96 | 0.32 |
| 0.33 | 0.5 | 0.9 | 0.7 | 3 | 0.14 | 0.6 | 0.065 |
| 0.5 | 1 | 0.75 | 0.75 | 3 | 0.33 | 0.75 | 0.25 |
| 0.1 | 0.11 | 0.95 | 0.95 | 19 | 0.05 | 0.68 | 0.006 |
| 0.02 | 0.02 | 0.8 | 0.6 | 2 | 0.33 | 0.04 | 0.007 |
| 0.1 | 0.11 | 0.85 | 0.5 | 1.7 | 0.3 | 0.16 | 0.032 |

*LR,* Likelihood ratio; *LR+,* positive likelihood ratio; *LR−,* negative likelihood ratio.

- Convert back to probability using the following formula:

$$\frac{\text{Odds}}{(1 + \text{Odds})}$$

*Example:* Odds of 1.3 is a probability of $1.3 \div (1 + 1.3) = 0.57$ (that is, 57%). Odds of 0.2 is a probability of $0.2 \div (1 + 0.2) = 0.17$.

## Putting It All Together: Decision Analysis

Thus far readers have developed the skills necessary to calculate an AT for the treatment at hand, estimate the pretest likelihood of the disease in question, and calculate the effect that the test would have on the current likelihood estimate. This information is all that is necessary to help the patient make the best decision possible.

The possible decision options the physician might face in typical clinical situation can be summarized with three words—*observe, treat,* and *test.* For clarity, *observe* means to decide against the definitive treatment (although the physician might choose to provide reassurance or symptomatic or supportive measures). *Treat* means to provide the specific treatment for the disease in question. *Test* means to defer the decision pending the test result and then to act accordingly. The three terms are described in more detail as follows:

1. **Observe:** The physician simply may forego testing and treatment and observe the patient.

   *Example:* A nonsmoking patient demonstrates a recent mild cough without physical findings and asks whether she needs a chest x-ray scan for lung cancer. You know that the disease the patient is asking about is so unlikely that testing would be abnormal only rarely. In addition, you determine, if the test happened to show an incidental minor abnormality, you probably would not act on it.

2. **Treat:** The physician may treat the patient without bothering to test.

   *Example:* A patient calls you and reports classic symptoms of a urinary infection with no complications or unusual risks. After performing a careful history, you prescribe a short course of antibiotics without bothering to perform a urine culture or analysis.

3. **Test:** The physician may decide to forego a decision until obtaining a test result. If the test is positive, the physician would choose to treat; if negative, observation would be the choice.

   *Example:* A patient comes to you with recent respiratory symptoms, a fever of 39.5° C and a productive cough. You hear abnormal lung sounds on your examination and decide to order a chest x-ray. If the test is normal, you decide to treat the patient symptomatically only. However, if it shows signs of pneumonia, you decide to treat the patient with an appropriate antibiotic.

Figure 4.6 illustrates these steps graphically. In it, the *observe* scenario refers to the top bar. *Treat* is shown in the second bar, and *test* is addressed in the lower two bars (one for when the pretest likelihood moves from above to below the AT and the other for when that likelihood moves from below to above the AT).

To summarize, if the testing might alter the pretest likelihood to a level that crosses the AT (that is, moves from above to below the AT or vice versa), the test is worth doing. If not, simple treatment or observation are recommended, depending on where the pretest likelihood lies.

**Real-World Nuances**  Stating that the mathematic representations presented previously are suited perfectly to actual practice would be naive. The important humanistic and nonquantitative elements that lend richness and complexity to medical practice also have profound effects on the decision-making process. One example of such an element is the "need-to-know" issue ("value of knowing") addressed previously.

**Handling "Wrong" Decision Requests by Patients**  Patients frequently visit the physician with expectations based on misinformation, previous medical experience, or other factors. Despite the physicians' attempts to explain their recommendations to the contrary, many patients may seem unconvinced or even skeptical. The physician then is torn between a desire to reassure and satisfy the patient's agenda and the need to do what best serves the patient's health needs. The following discussion may provide physicians with some "immunization" to help them respond to such situations.

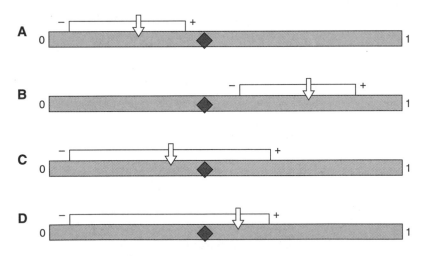

**Figure 4.6**  Four decision scenarios depicting the possible impact of a diagnostic test on a decision about whether to observe only **(A)**, treat without testing **(B)**, test and decide when the pretest likelihood is below the AT **(C)**, or test and decide when the pretest likelihood is above the AT **(D)**.

***Request for an inappropriate test*** If the inappropriate test that the patient requests is inexpensive and free of risk, a wise approach to this situation is to agree to perform the test after explaining the risk of false-positive and false-negative results. Next, the physician can allow the patient to decide explicitly in advance what that patient would do in the case of both a positive result and a negative result. Sometimes the very process of sorting out these options may help the patient realize why the physician does not advise the test in question.

For example, I have encountered this patient response with the prostate-specific antigen (PSA) test currently available, particularly by young men at low risk for prostate cancer. Patients request the PSA test, often recounting personal experiences, such as "My neighbor had one, and it showed cancer; they removed his prostate and saved his life." Most patients at normal risk for cancer demonstrate normal results. However, some individuals may demonstrate results that are mildly positive, the vast majority of which are falsely positive. If a patient then proceeds with the usual subsequent evaluation, that individual must undergo a painful set of prostate biopsies, with a small but clear risk of complications. When early prostate cancer is detected, the evidence is unclear as to the benefits of treatment, and its risks include impotence and urinary incontinence. Furthermore, whether treatment at this earliest state of disease even improves outcomes remains unclear; many such individuals may have lived decades with inapparent cancer and died of another disease even without treatment.

Following is a description that illustrates one approach to the situation in which the patient requests an inappropriate PSA test against the physician's recommendation:

**Example**

"I'd be happy to perform this test, Mr. Smith, but before deciding, you should be aware that the test is imperfect. In men like you, in whom the risk of having prostate cancer is quite low, the scientific research shows that PSA fails to detect most early cancers, and more importantly, many patients who turn up positive do not have cancer at all. Unfortunately, the only way to know this is to perform a biopsy. This test involves the insertion of an instrument into the rectum, and the passage of a needle through the rectum into the prostate several times. In addition, whether the type of prostate cancer found with this approach even benefits from early treatment is unclear.

"So if you choose to have me perform the test, you should be prepared for what a positive result might involve and the uncertainties it carries. Now, would you like to proceed with it or perhaps give it some thought so that we can talk about it next time?"

Several points of interest are covered in the previous example. First, the physician does not refuse to perform the test but simply educates the patient as to why it may not be a good idea. Second, the physician demonstrates respect for the patient's values by presenting the facts and asking the patient to weigh the possibilities. True, the wording in the example may paint an unappealing picture, but the advice is accurate. The physician's explanation also provides advice in the unlikely event of a positive result so that the patient will not be taken by surprise. If the patient persists in the request, the physician can perform the test, knowing not only that the result most likely will be normal but also taking solace in the fact that the patient is well informed.

Another point worth noting in the previous example is how the physician avoids specific numbers. Some patients may require specifics, but my experience shows that thoughtful use of phrases such as *quite a few, many,* and *most* are sufficient in most cases. The physician's challenge is to be true to the evidence in word choice, even if actual numbers are not discussed.

After reviewing the evidence, readers may construct such responses to common situations in the context of their own experiences in which patients have requested unnecessary treatments. These sample responses should serve most practitioners well; rather than receiving each such request as a frustrating challenge, instead such requests can be opportunities for physicians to educate patients and affirm their own knowledge and decision skills.

*Request for an inappropriate treatment* Although a patient's request for inappropriate treatment is superficially a treatment rather than a diagnosis issue, in effect it includes both components because it revolves around the likelihood of a disease. The classic example involves a patient requesting antibiotics for an uncomplicated viral upper respiratory infection. ("I know it's strep/sinusitis/bronchitis.") A physician who practices EBDM may address the problem as in the following example.

| Example |

"Yes, Bob, with those nasty symptoms I can see why you wondered about sinusitis, but based on my findings this diagnosis seems very unlikely. The problem with antibiotics is that once in a while they have side effects that can make you more ill than you are now, and they usually don't help very much anyway. In fact, the evidence suggests that in situations such as this, the risk of side effects is greater than any benefit you might gain from the drug.

"Why don't we try this strategy. I'd like to try this powerful decongestant for a few days. If in 3 or 4 days you have not noticed any improvement or if your symptoms worsen before then, give me a call and we can decide what to do at that time."

Key points in the previous example include acknowledgment of the legitimacy of the patient's request. Also, laying out the outcomes in terms of the risk exceeding the benefits makes the logic of the decision more explicit. A compromise approach that leaves the door open to possible reconsideration is a technique that placates many patients. Finally, the physician's use of an alternative "powerful" prescription medication (perhaps little more effective than a placebo, but in any case affirming the treatment-worthy nature of the patient's symptoms) can be helpful.

Experienced physicians know that the previous situations can occur in an infinite number of variations. These sample dialogues are examples of how the physician can turn a request for inappropriate care into an opportunity for the use of EBDM and communication with the patient, as opposed to the practitioner's "caving in" to the patient's request and possibly doing the wrong thing. Clearly not all patients can be satisfied by even the best explanations, but the right phrase that uses the right evidence is the best approach.

**Special Case: Screening Tests**  To qualify as screenable a disease should meet specific criteria including the following:[7]

- The disease must be common enough to warrant the cost and effort of screening.
- An accurate screening test must be available for patients in the preclinical stage of the disease.
- An effective treatment must be available that is more beneficial when applied before the disease becomes clinically apparent than after it is apparent.

Screening tests, such as mammography and fecal occult blood, are nothing more than diagnostic tests in the setting of a very low likelihood of disease. The prevalence or pretest likelihood is typically in the range of 1% to 2%. (For example, colon neoplasm and fecal occult blood testing presume a pretest likelihood of approximately 1.1%.[1])

These low-likelihood settings have unfortunate effects on the interpretation of diagnostic tests, even extremely accurate ones. For example, a screenable disease has a prevalence of 1:1000 (human immunodeficiency virus [HIV] in military inductees, for instance). In addition, a very fine diagnostic test has both a sensitivity and specificity of 99% (such as the HIV enzyme-linked immunosorbent assay [ELISA] antibody tests). Figure 4.7 illustrates how this situation would unfold.

Experienced practitioners often appreciate this effect (the large number of false positives in screening tests). For example, a large number of women endure breast biopsies for abnormal mammograms and end up with benign lesions; in addition, a large number of colonoscopies for fecal occult blood fail to show cancer or precancerous lesions.

A similar effect occurs when the physician orders automated panels of blood tests rather than focused, specific tests. The "extra" unintended tests essentially act as screening tests in healthy individuals; these tests look for diseases that the physician has no reason to suspect. Added to the fact that the normal range for each test probably preordains that 10% of normal individuals will have abnormal results, the finding of even one individual with a completely normal multiphasic blood test panel seems surprising.

Lest the practitioner become cynical about the value of screening tests (although cynicism concerning multiphasic test panels is permissible), the ten-

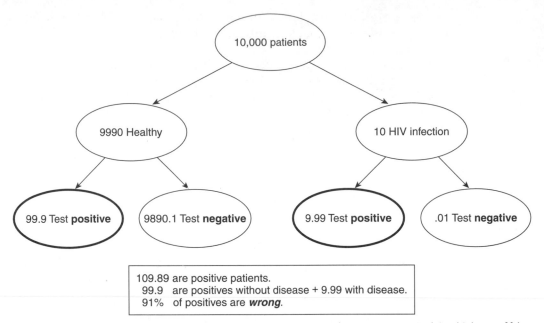

**Figure 4.7**    In low-likelihood situations such as screening, even extremely accurate tests result in a high rate of false positives. *HIV,* Human immunodeficiency virus.

dency in recent years has favored a highly selective approach. Most positive results initiate a second set of confirmatory tests rather than direct treatment (for example, HIV by Western blot technique). Increasingly, screening tests are confined to high-risk populations to reduce the false-positivity rate. Furthermore, many physicians are educating their patients more accurately about the implications of positive screening tests; that is, such tests are presented as "red flags" requiring follow-up rather than as definitive evidence of disease. Still, a healthy level of humility about the limitations of screening of healthy patients is warranted.

## SUMMARY

This chapter focuses on the ideal view of testing as a means to refine the estimate of the likelihood of a disease. The importance of a reasonably accurate pretest likelihood estimate is emphasized. Test evidence consists of sensitivity and specificity, both of which are used to calculate LRs. Given the pretest likelihood and the LR, the practitioner can calculate mentally the posttest likelihood of disease.

Strategies used to search the literature for sound evidence about testing are presented with the now-familiar two-pass strategy. Once found, the evidence can be appraised for suitability by use of several criteria about its applicability and validity.

A test's decision value depends on its ability to alter the pretest likelihood to a level that crosses the AT, either by lowering it from above to below or raising it from below to above the AT. This technique allows the practitioner to decide in advance whether to simply observe the patient, test and decide about the treatment in question according to the test results, or treat the patient immediately without bothering to perform the test.

Finally, the special cases of screening tests and multiphasic test panels are discussed, with an emphasis on the high false-positive rate inherent in very low pretest likelihood situations.

## REFERENCES

1. Allison JE and others: A comparison of fecal occult-blood tests for colorectal-cancer screening, *N Engl J Med* 334:155-159, 1996.
2. Gabriel SE and others: The use of clinical characteristics to predict the results of temporal artery biopsy among patients with suspected giant cell arteritis. *J Rheumatol* 22(1):93-96, 1995.
3. Jaeschke R and others, for the Evidence-Based Medicine Working Group: Users' guides to the medical literature. III. How to use an article about a diagnostic test. A: Are the results of the study valid? *JAMA* 271:389-391, 1994.
4. Jaeschke R and others, for the Evidence-Based Medicine Working Group: Users' guides to the medical literature. III. How to use an article about a diagnostic test. B: What are the results and will they help me in caring for my patients? *JAMA* 271:703-707, 1994.
5. Robb-Nicholson C and others: Diagnostic value of the history and examination in giant cell arteritis: a clinical pathological study of 81 temporal artery biopsies, *J Rheumatol* 15(12):1793-1796, 1988.
6. Sox HC and others: *Medical decision making*, Stoneham, Mass, 1988, Butterworth-Heinemann.
7. U.S. Preventive Services Task Force: *Guide to clinical preventive services*, ed 2, Baltimore, 1996, Williams & Wilkins.
8. Valdimarsson T and others: Is small bowel biopsy necessary in adults with suspected celiac disease and igA anti-endomysium antibodies? 100% positive predictive value for celiac disease in adults, *Dig Dis Sci* 41(1):83-87, 1996.

# CHAPTER 5

# *Risk*

## INTRODUCTION

Risk is the potential of an exposure to cause in increase in the frequency or intensity of an undesirable outcome. The exposure may take many forms, ranging from unavoidable factors, such as gender or age, to potentially avoidable ones, such as tobacco use or excessive solar radiation. The terms *harm* and *etiology* are used sometimes in the same context.

Chapter 1 already discussed one type of risk—side effects from medical treatment, which were referred to in that discussion as *harm,* with the presumption of an offsetting benefit. In that context the physician usually can quantify the degree of risk prospectively using a randomized controlled trial (RCT). Because these risks often are accepted ethically and socially as a trade-off for the potential benefits of the treatment, such studies are practical, ethical, and necessary.

This chapter focuses on the type of risks the physician cannot often study in the same way treatments are studied—unintended risks that are not the result of treatment and often are intrinsic to the environment or lifestyle of a population. Generally the goal of research into risks is to identify those that were unrecognized or unproved previously. Because such studies often contain many confounding variables, risk identification is a challenging task.

# *Components of Risk Decisions*

## UNDERSTANDING THE NUMERIC PARAMETERS OF RISK

The terms *absolute risk* and *relative risk* were discussed in Chapter 1 in the context of either disease or treatment outcomes. They are summarized briefly in the following section. The remaining parameter this discussion aims to describe at length is known as the *odds ratio*.

In the definitions that follow the term *control event rate* (CER) means the rate of an outcome in the control or unexposed (risk-free) population. The term *exposed event rate* (EER, which is similar to the experimental event rate) refers to the population that was exposed to the risk.

### Absolute Risk

Absolute risk (AR) is the difference between the rate of the EER and CER expressed as absolute percentage points (EER − CER). It describes the number of percentage points by which the probability of the outcome in the exposed group exceeds its probability in the control group.

### Relative Risk

Relative risk (RR) is the ratio of the EER to the CER (EER ÷ CER). It describes the risk in the exposed group as a proportion of the risk in the unexposed group. The RR in question is relative to the absolute baseline risk in the unexposed group.

### Number Needed to Harm

Number needed to harm (NNH) is analogous to number needed to treat (NNT) and is calculated as 100 ÷ AR. It describes the number of individuals who need to be exposed to a risk on average for one individual to develop the undesirable outcome. Given the NNH alone the physician can calculate the AR by inverting the equation: AR = 100 ÷ NNH.

### Odds Ratios: Reporting Case-Control Studies

If all studies of risk were cohort studies or RCTs, little need would exist to express the results other than as ARs and RRs. However, many risk factors are either too dangerous to study ethically in a prospective manner or produce an effect so small that enormous cohorts would be required to achieve statistical validity. For example, to detect the risk of nonsteroidal agents in individuals with end-stage renal failure, a study's researchers would have to follow a cohort of 1 million individuals for more than 2 years![2]

The alternative to such an impractical study is the case-control design, which is discussed in the following section. Odds ratios are the common parameter generated by such studies. Because odds ratios are understood more readily if the reader is familiar with the case-control methodology, the discussion focuses on the research design first, as opposed to the previous chapters' discussions, which focused on the parameters and then on the study design.

CHAPTER 5   **SECTION TWO**

# *Evidence about Risk*

## UNDERSTANDING CLINICAL STUDIES ABOUT RISK

If a risk is considered "acceptable" to an informed and competent patient as part of a clinical trial, its study may assume the form of either an RCT or a cohort study, both of which are discussed in detail in Chapter 3. Consider a few examples.

*Example*

Individuals who drink three or more cups of coffee a day are enrolled in a cohort study, along with similar subjects who do not drink coffee. Because the subjects are not asked to change their behavior in any way, the researchers may consider it acceptable that the subjects remain unaware of their hypothesis that coffee helps cause pancreatic cancer. The subjects are followed closely enough to determine the incidence of pancreatic cancer over 5 years. This design is a prospective cohort study.

*Example*

Subjects are informed that the study in which they are enrolled is designed to assess risk factors for osteoarthritis. Of a sedentary population, one group is assigned randomly to a swimming cohort, another to a jogging cohort, and a third to a walking cohort. The hypothesis, unknown to the participants, is that jogging causes osteoarthritis. The exercise regimens are supervised over 5 years, after which all subjects are assessed blindly for signs and symptoms of osteoarthritis. Because several potential risks are introduced randomly, the risks are controlled, and the researchers are at least single-blinded, this design describes an RCT of a risk factor.

In such studies the results would be reported as AR and RR. Unfortunately, many risks are unacceptable or uncontrollable. For example, a physician is among the first to see several patients with cases of mesothelioma (a dangerous cancer of the lining of various body cavities) in workers exposed to asbestos. The practitioner decides to study this phenomenon both rigorously and ethically. Is the asbestos the cause? Is the population of employees working in the plant at inherently high risk for this disease due to common ancestry, water supply, or some other occult factor?

Furthermore, cohort and RCT designs cannot always be used for risk research because many risks cause only small increases in the feared outcome. For example, some 10,000 subjects in each group would be required to demonstrate an AR of 0.01% with an acceptable 95% confidence interval! Yet such an increase may have great importance if the risk were a common environmental exposure. Many risks take decades to manifest their consequences; a 20-year cohort study, although possible, presents significant logistic challenges. For these reasons the practitioner who seeks to study the workers exposed to asbestos may see a case-control study as the only reasonable approach. Such studies have become more frequent recently.

In summary, three factors create the need to use a case-control study design, as follows:

1. Rarity of the outcome in the populations to be studied
2. Ethical concerns about intentional exposure of a population to a potentially dangerous risk (as distinct from study of a population already exposed to the risk in their customary lifestyle)
3. Necessity for long-term exposure before effects become apparent, leading to impracticality of prospective designs

## Case-Control Study Design

A case-control study starts with individuals *who already have developed the undesirable outcome* suspected of being caused by a risk exposure. Thus the prevalence of the outcome in this population is 100%. The next step is to identify a second population whose members do not have the outcome in question but who otherwise are as similar as possible to the afflicted population. The researcher then determines as accurately as possible the frequency of exposure to the suspected risk in each population. Case-control studies measure retrospectively the likelihood of a risk factor given the presence of disease (comparable to the sensitivity of a diagnostic test, which measures the likelihood of an abnormal result given the presence of disease).

**Weaknesses of Case-Control Methodology**  Case-control studies have practical advantages, as discussed previously. Unfortunately, they are more vulnerable to bias than are cohort studies or RCTs.

In constructing the populations for a case-control study, the researchers postulate that risk R causes disease D. They attempt to isolate disease D as the *only* identifiable difference between the control group (whose members do *not* have disease D) and the case group (whose members *do* have disease D). This task is daunting because accounting for all lifestyle variables is almost never achievable. The goal is to ensure all participants represent the well-characterized baseline population, with only disease D to distinguish them from one another.

In the asbestos example the control group may be co-workers in the same factory as the aforementioned mesothelioma patients—but those whose job descriptions do not expose them to asbestos. Finding such matched populations can be challenging because the researcher has to assume *a priori* that the suspected risk is indeed the cause; if the cause turns out to be something else for which the "matched" population fails to account, the researcher may falsely ascribe the risk to asbestos, when it may be due to some other occult factor. Furthermore, the afflicted population may be far more likely to *recall* a risk exposure in the enrollment survey than those who are free of disease. These factors represent just some of the potential pitfalls of case selection.

In a *population-based* case-control study, these pitfalls are addressed by selection of the representative base population in advance, followed by identification of those individuals within it who have or do not have the disease. (That is, both groups are drawn from the same initially identified population.) Compared with groups assembled from, for instance, consecutive hospital admissions, the population-based study represents a better chance that the findings will be valid; admitted patients do not represent the general population and by definition have important unrelated health conditions that can bias the results.

**Bias Due to Disease Duration**  When feasible, the outcomes best considered are those of recent onset; long-standing effects make identification of remote contaminating variables even more difficult. In addition, a risk factor can cause a disease of spontaneous etiology to last longer rather than actually causing the disease (for example, sinusitis in a population of smokers compared to non-smokers). In that case, over time patients can accumulate in a group's prevalence population because they remain sick longer than those individuals with the same disease in the unexposed population, a factor that can generate results that incorrectly reflect a cause and effect.

**Recall and Measurement Bias**  A final pitfall in case-control design is that the disease itself can affect the very exposure being studied, or at least the measurement of it. For example, researchers design a study to determine whether individuals with staphylococcal blood infection are more likely to have suffered a recent skin wound (as a potential entry point for bacteria). First, patients admitted for staphylococcal infections may comb their memories far more meticulously than individuals in a control population and thus may recall such injuries more readily, a concept known as *recall bias*. Second, the examiners of such patients may perform far more thorough physical exams for possible skin wounds than they would perform in otherwise healthy individuals, a concept known as *measurement bias*. Finally, the illness may cause the patients to confine themselves to home or bed in the days preceding admission, leading to a lower likelihood of spontaneous skin injury than that in the control group.

**Matching within a Case-Control Study**  Sometimes researchers attempt to strengthen the design by matching cases to controls on a paired basis, ensuring that at least age, gender, clinical status, and other similar factors are comparable. In this design, cases are compared with their controls, which are matched by age, gender, or other factors, and the results are aggregated on a pair-by-pair basis (not on a group-to-group basis). Although this action can help reduce the likelihood of bias caused by the variables that were matched intentionally, it introduces the risk that the *intentional* matching may cause *unintentional* matching. For instance, if one of the intentionally matched characteristics is associated occultly with the likelihood of true risk exposure, the importance of that exposure may be obscured.

A study seeks to determine whether sun exposure is associated with skin cancer. The older an individual, the greater the lifetime sun exposure and the greater the risk. Therefore older persons have a greater risk than younger ones.

A case-control study pairs subjects by age, and its results demonstrate no difference between the two groups (younger and older). Through a focus on pairing, the fact that age is associated with sun exposure is masked, and the sun-cancer link thus is missed.

**Case-Control Design Conclusions**  Case-control studies allow for the investigation of phenomena beyond the reach of prospective designs because of practical, statistical, and ethical considerations. Although methodologically more prone to bias than cohort studies and RCTs, case-control studies are performed frequently. The results often are reported as odds ratios, the focus of the following section.

## Odds Ratios Revisited

Odds ratios reflect the *odds* of a risk exposure in the case group divided by the *odds* of exposure in the control group in a case-control study. Readers may note the similarity between odds ratios and RR; the only arithmetic difference is that the former is a ratio of two odds, whereas the latter is a ratio of two probabilities.

Examine, for example, a hypothetical population with a disease prevalence of 5% for individuals in whom a risk factor is absent, and 20% for individuals in whom the risk factor is present; the risk factors increase the likelihood of the disease fourfold. Assume that 25% of the population overall is exposed to the risk. Researchers, of course, do not know these numbers and seek to discover them by examining the data. The only information they have is a suspicion that the risk causes the disease in some individuals.

Figure 5.1 illustrates the way in which 1000 such individuals might distribute themselves. The researcher comes along *after* the fact and sees only the information contained in the two rectangular boxes at the bottom of the figure. The researcher describes one group of individuals with a disease and certain prevalence of the risk factor and another group without the disease and with a lower prevalence of the risk factor. As shown, this information enables the researcher to calculate an odds ratio as follows:

$$\frac{\text{Risk present} \div \text{risk absent [case group]}}{\text{Risk present} \div \text{risk absent [control group]}}$$

where the numerator refers to the case group and the denominator to the control group.

The advantage of the odds ratio is that it does not depend on either the baseline prevalence of the risk factor or the absolute incidence of the disease, factors

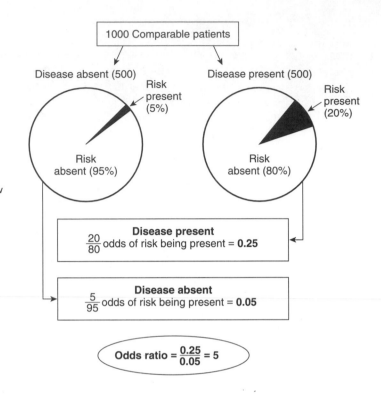

**Figure 5.1** Step-by-step breakdown of how odds ratios are derived in a case-control study.

that after all are not evident from the case-control data (but which the researcher may learn from a subsequent cross-sectional study* of the population).

Perhaps the researcher prefers probability to odds; why not use a "prevalence ratio" instead through comparison of the *probability* of risk exposure in the sick group of individuals to that of the healthy group (a sort of RR) from these data? The issue has been discussed in the literature,[1] and the answer is provided in Table 5.1.

If a risk causes disease with a certain "power," then no reason exists why that power should vary with the prevalence of the risk in the population in question. True, the higher the prevalence of the risk factor, the greater the number of subjects who develop the disease, but the inherent danger of the risk to any given exposed individual is independent of the number of others exposed.

Table 5.1 demonstrates that the whimsical "prevalence ratio" varies with the underlying prevalence of the risk in the population in question while the odds ratio remains the same no matter how much the risk prevalence varies. The odds ratio can be calculated without knowledge of the risk prevalence.

---

*A cross-sectional study is a mere "snapshot" of a population used to determine its status at a single point in time; it is a detailed quantitative description. Some data it provides include the prevalence (*not* the incidence) of a disease, risk factor exposures, and demographic information.

**TABLE 5.1**
Comparison of Risk-Exposure Likelihood in Two Groups

| Baseline Risk Prevalence | Healthy Population with Risk Present (%) | Sick Population with Risk Present (%) | Prevalence Ratio* | Odds Ratio† |
|---|---|---|---|---|
| 10 | 8.6 | 31 | 3.6 | 4.75 |
| 25 | 22 | 57 | 2.6 | 4.75 |
| 50 | 46 | 80 | 1.8 | 4.75 |
| 75 | 72 | 92 | 1.3 | 4.75 |

*Probability.
†Odds.

The main point in this discussion is that in a case-control study, the researcher should not look at the comparative probabilities of risk in the two groups but rather at the odds ratio.*

Statisticians have cautioned that although conceptualizing an odds ratio as similar to an RR is tempting, this comparison is acceptable only when the risk is low (for example, less than 1%).† Statistical corrections for the use of probability do exist, but they are beyond the scope of this discussion.[6] In general, the practitioner can use an odds ratio in the same way an RR is used within this lower prevalence range.

> **Example**
>
> A case-control study shows that the odds ratio of more than 3 hours of sun exposure per day for development of melanoma of the skin is 4. If the unexposed population has an incidence of melanoma of 0.5%, an exposed population would be expected to have an incidence of 0.5% × 4, or 2%. If the unexposed population had an incidence of 15%, the practitioner would not rely on odds ratios in this manner because this value is well above the 1% range mentioned in the previous paragraph.

**Adjusted Odds Ratios** Consider the following example involving adjustments in odds ratios.

> **Example**
>
> Suppose you decide to study alcohol as a risk for esophageal cancer. You follow two groups comparable except in their alcohol use. Despite your

---

*This situation is analogous to the use of predictive values and likelihood ratios; the former is valid only at a specific pretest likelihood, whereas the latter can be used with any pretest likelihood. Similarly, odds ratios are applicable at any risk prevalence.

†This case is seen frequently for environmental or lifestyle risks; in fact, the risks usually are far lower than 1%.

best efforts, tobacco use is slightly higher in the control group than in the alcohol-using group. Because tobacco is a known risk factor for esophageal cancer, you decide this factor may obscure alcohol's risk potential by disproportionately amplifying the risk in the control group.

When such a confounder (that is, tobacco use as a risk for esophageal cancer) is well characterized in the medical literature, statisticians can correct for it by performing internal analyses across both study groups to assess the importance of the imbalanced risk distribution. Based on that measurement, they can "adjust" the odds ratio for alcohol use to correct ostensibly for the effect of the uneven tobacco use between the groups. This correction is known as the *adjusted odds ratio*. Although a theoretically valid tool, adjusted odds ratios may provoke questions about statistical validity if the subgroups being divided do not contain large numbers of subjects. The details of this issue are beyond the scope of this discussion, but suffice it to say that if a study fails to show an important risk based on unadjusted odds ratios, demonstrating the risk solely with *adjusted* odds ratios, some skepticism is warranted. Usually, unless the two cohorts somehow contain a very "nonrandom" allocation of participants, the adjusted odds ratios simply reinforce a risk already demonstrated with the unadjusted numbers.

**Hazard Ratios** Generated by a statistical technique known as *Cox proportionate hazard analysis,* a hazard ratio is a refinement of the odds ratio, typically applied when the outcome is mortality. When death of a study's subjects is caused by the presence of a risk factor, the number of participants within the cohort dwindles as the study continues.

Suppose a risk factor is associated with an RR of survival at 1 year of 0.75 (that is, 75% of exposed subjects surviving, relative to the otherwise comparable unexposed individuals). Now, at 1 year, only 75% of the original risk cohort remains in the study (the control group remaining nearly intact at its original complement of participants). This shrunken contingent does not carry as much statistical weight as the original 100% group. At 2 years, only 90 participants may remain in the control group and 52 in the risk group. Again the statistical meaningfulness of these numbers changes. The hazard analysis corrects for this dynamic situation, applying a "smoothing" correction for the inevitable fluctuation of the numbers over time. With the indulgence of their statistician colleagues for this undoubtedly gross oversimplification, medical practitioners may remain content with conceptualizing hazard ratios as similar to odds ratios—but with these corrections applied.

## Cohort Studies for Risk Assessment

Notwithstanding the common necessity of reliance on case-control studies for risks, prospective cohort studies can be achieved in certain situations. These instances rely on the effect of natural exposures on some populations and not on others. For instance, smokers and nonsmokers, diabetic and nondiabetic individuals, and communities near Chernobyl and those distant from it all exist. If all factors other than the risk being studied are the same (an ideal not achieved easily), any differences in the outcome of interest are assumed to be due to the exposure.

Cohort studies are prospective, a major strength. A population containing both unexposed and exposed individuals is identified from the natural setting, and subjects are assessed for the criteria the researchers deem appropriate. Especially important are those factors aside from the risk being studied that might affect the key outcomes—that is, those that might "contaminate" the results. If subjects are excluded for any reason, such exclusion is done best by an examiner who is unaware of the subjects' risk exposure status (the equivalent of concealment in an RCT). At the outset, subjects are allocated into those who are exposed to the risk (risk positive) and those who are not (risk negative).

Over time as the groups are followed, some subjects presumably develop the outcome of interest. Researchers remain blind to the risk status whenever possible, and sometimes the subjects can be blinded as well. On completion of the study the two groups are compared.

Included in the inherent vulnerability of this type of study is the inability of the researchers to identify all other factors possibly associated with risk status. For example, do nonsmokers also exercise more? Do individuals in high radon-gas zip codes also earn more money than those in low radon-gas areas? Identified or suspected factors can be dealt with in the analysis. The *unidentified* factors are those that always raise issues of a study's credibility (that is, validity).

## Results of Cohort Studies of Risk

The statistics underlying a large cohort study can be ponderous. Logistic regression and multivariate analysis are examples of techniques that aim to isolate one effect to specific variables by weighing or correcting for the effects of others. Detailing the complexities of the tools is beyond the scope of this discussion, but such tools are necessary features of most cohort studies of risk. Landmark projects, such as the Framingham cardiovascular risk study, attest to the potential importance of such evidence.

A cohort study generally is preferable to a case-control study, all other factors aside. Practitioners should seek them out for risk evidence.

# RETRIEVING EVIDENCE ABOUT RISK

## Master Evidence Question

The Master Evidence Question for risk is as follows:

> *Do subjects exposed to risk have a higher incidence of outcome compared with subjects not exposed?*

The evidence may be found as AR, RR, or odds ratio. As always, the first step to obtain such evidence is to search preappraised data repositories, such as

Best Evidence. If the results are insufficient, MEDLINE should be the next stop.

The two-pass strategy for risk evidence is used to unearth the most relevant evidence available. (The two-pass strategy concept is introduced and explained in detail in Chapter 3 in the section about evidence retrieval.) The strategy is based on the 1994 article by Haynes,[4] with modifications to reflect search-engine improvements. An example of a search strategy involving risk follows, with examples of actual search criteria.

**Pass 1:** Risk words AND outcome words AND (risk OR odds ratio)
*Example:* caffeine AND pancreatic cancer AND (risk OR odds ratio)

**Pass 2:** Pass 1 AND (cohort OR case control)
*Example:* #1 AND (cohort OR case control)

Users should recall the use of the wild-card character; omitting it enables medical subject heading (MeSH) explosion and phrase matching, whereas using it matches derivative terms but suppresses the MeSH and phrase-matching features. Consider the following example.

---
*Example*
---

You consider studying the following effects: Is coffee ingestion a risk for pancreatic cancer? *or* What is the risk of pancreatic cancer in coffee users compared with nonusers?

**Pass 1:** coffee AND pancreatic cancer AND (risk OR odds ratio)
*Results:* 89

**Pass 2:** #1 AND (cohort OR case control)
*Results:* 49

The previous example turns up numerous citations, including several applicable ones and several with apparently rigorous methodology. A detailed review of selected articles suggests that coffee ingestion and pancreatic cancer are not associated.

## JUDGING THE SUITABILITY OF RISK EVIDENCE

### Assessing Applicability

The applicability of risk evidence is appraised in much the same way as most types of evidence are appraised—determination of whether the patient in question could have been included among the subjects in the study. In addition to the usual biographic, gender, and lifestyle variables that require comparison, some additional criteria questions apply.

### Are the Duration and Intensity of Exposure Similar to Those of My Patient?

A study of intense radon exposure for 10 years may not apply to a patient who recently learned that the rarely used basement of her new house contains low levels of radon.

### Is My Patient's Environment Equally Free of Potential Contaminating Variables or Exposures?

Example

> If the incidence of lung cancer reportedly was increased among smokers who also work in coal mines, the study's information may not apply to nonsmokers who work in coal mines.

For a case-control study, determination of whether the groups are applicable to the patient in question may prove difficult. Often the subjects are drawn from hospital admissions or other groups that may represent narrow populations. For example, the study of edema as a risk factor for development of deep vein thrombosis (DVT, a large blood clot in the leg) includes DVT patients in the case group, whereas the control group members consist of other admissions with a wide range of alternative diagnoses. Are the results of this study applicable to an active outpatient with edema? A much better design for this scenario would be a population-based study containing a large group of active outpatients, from which a group with recently diagnosed DVT was selected (the case group) and compared with a comparable group from the same population whose members did not have DVT.

## Assessing Validity

Perhaps to a greater degree than with other types of studies, assessment of the validity of a case-control study is a complex and challenging task. This is one instance in which physicians are well advised to consult expert commentators and editorial boards. A physician who wants to assess the validity of a case-control study or assess whether the editorial board members have performed and interpreted the study correctly must become acquainted with several issues. These issues are summarized in the following six questions:

1. Are the two groups (case and control) similar except concerning disease status?
2. Were the groups selected from a predefined population of interest?
3. Were both the risk status and the disease status measured identically in both groups?
4. Was the duration of the risk exposure adequate and similar in both groups?
5. Might the disease itself have affected the likelihood of risk exposure? For example, a sedentary lifestyle may be a risk factor for a disease that itself

affects mobility. Clarify whether the reported "risk" actually may be an effect of the disease it is said to "cause."

6. Was the case group structured to capture primarily diseases of recent onset? If not, does data demonstrate similar odds ratios for recent and chronic victims? Is the disease rapidly fatal or brief in duration, in which situation the case group should focus on incidence and not prevalence?

That case-control studies generate large volumes of "letters to the editor" (that is, controversy) attests to the difficulty in their appraisal. Rarely does a study fulfill all the previously stated criteria, and even if it does, specific issues often are raised that question the study's validity. The best approach for a non-expert appraiser is to derive a general sense of a study's validity standards, read the editors' comments, if available, and accept all conclusions derived solely from a case-control study as less than definitive. Figure 5.2 summarizes the steps used to appraise an article involving risk in general.

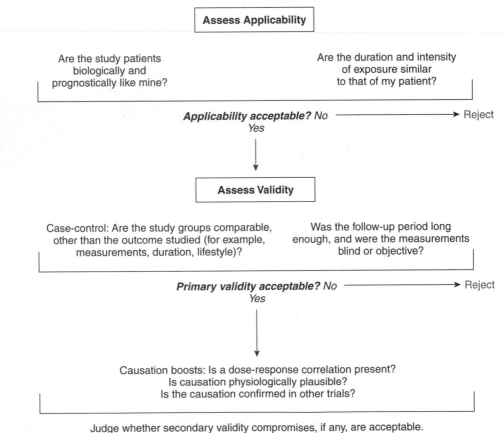

**Figure 5.2**  Appraisal of risk evidence from case-control studies. Note that *accept* and *reject* are two extremes of inference as to how closely a study approximates the "truth." The practitioner's interpretation generally falls somewhere between the two extremes.

## Association and Causation

A valid risk study, especially a cohort study or an RCT, can establish a clear *association* between an exposure and an outcome. Before assuming the existence of a cause-and-effect relationship, however, the practitioner should apply further scrutiny. For instance, risk A is associated with risk B, and risk B causes outcome 1. A study might identify a valid association between risk A and outcome 1—risk A possibly being a marker for risk B, which is the true cause of outcome 1. The problem in this assumption is that removal of risk A from the environment does not affect the frequency of the outcome. When a remedy or preventive intervention for the risk factor is implemented, the true agent generally must be identified. These additional observations help strengthen the causation hypothesis, as illustrated in the following questions:

1. Is a dose-response correlation present? If higher levels of risk exposure cause more disease than lower levels, this fact strengthens the causation hypothesis.
2. Is the timing consistent? Especially interesting to note is whether the outcome was on the wane before the reduction of the risk factor. If coronary deaths already were diminishing before the exercise boom, for example, this evidence would speak against inactivity as a cause for cardiovascular disease.
3. Does a biologically plausible explanation exist for causation? Although the lack of such plausibility simply may reflect the current lack of knowledge about the pathophysiology of the disease in question, alignment of basic science with the results can be reassuring to some practitioners.

# *Helping the Patient Decide*

## USING RISK EVIDENCE IN MEDICAL DECISIONS

### Master Decision Question

The Master Decision Question in risk scenarios is as follows:

*Given the known risk, does the potential reduction in risk consequences warrant the measures necessary to avoid the risk factor?*

In other words, is the hassle of removing the risk factor worth it? The first step is to estimate the patient's likelihood of disease with and without exposure to the risk.

### Using Absolute and Relative Risk to Estimate Postexposure Likelihood

If the patient in question happens to fall into the same profile as the members of a population reported in a suitable cohort study, the practitioner can use the AR reported in the study. RR can be used instead if the patient's baseline differs slightly from that described in the study.

| Example |

The risk of stroke due to carotid artery surgery in nonsmokers is reported to be 1%; in patients who smoke the risk of stroke from the surgery is 2%. Thus the AR is 1%, and the RR is 2.

Your patient is a smoker, but in your hospital the risk of stroke from this procedure is 0.75%. You use the RR of 2 to estimate the patient's risk in your hospital to be 2 × 0.75%, or 1.5%.

If the patient's risk is *substantially* different from that of the study population members, several problems arise. Other synergistic risk factors (for example, risk of coronary disease in sedentary, diabetic, nonsmoking individuals) may be reported, but if the patient is a diabetic smoker, the practitioner should be reluctant to apply that evidence because of applicability issues. The practitioner may be tempted to use RR by applying this value to the specific patient's higher baseline risk, for example. Unfortunately, the application of RR is not legitimate unless the baseline event rates (those in the study and in the patient) are fairly close.

| Example |

Consider a study that reports a 25% disease incidence in a control group and a 55% incidence in a risk-exposed group. The RR is 2.2.

If your patient's baseline risk is 27%, or even 30%, simple multiplication of the baseline by 2.2 to produce a prediction of the risk after exposure may be fairly accurate. However, suppose your patient's baseline risk is 50%. Multiplying this value by the RR of 2.2 produces greater than a

100% likelihood of disease, clearly an invalid result. The farther you stray from the reported baseline risk, the larger this distortion becomes.

AR and RR should be applied only when the practitioner estimates the patient's baseline risk to be close to that reported in the research (or at least has no reason to assume it is dissimilar).[5] Fortunately, such closely matched baseline results are often the case.

## Using Odds Ratios To Estimate Postexposure Likelihood

Although the validity of odds ratios (and hazard ratios) derived from case-control studies is considered weaker than evidence derived from cohort studies, odds ratios can be applied to any baseline risk, similar to RR when the baseline risk is low. Simply substituting the odds ratio for RR provides a quick estimate of the postexposure likelihood of the outcome.

When risk is higher than 1%, for example, the practitioner may apply odds ratios and risk analogous to their use with likelihood ratios and diagnostic tests; odds ratios can be used to calculate postexposure likelihood as follows:

$$\text{Postexposure odds} = \text{baseline odds} \times \text{odds ratio}$$

> *Example*
>
> A case-control study reveals an odds ratio of 4.75 for a certain chemical exposure as a risk for skin cancer.
>
> You learn from an independent, cross-sectional study that the odds of this skin cancer in your region are 1:199 (0.05%). You then can multiply the odds by 4.75 to calculate your postexposure odds of skin cancer: $(1 \div 199) \times 4.75 = 0.024$ odds = 2.3%. This low-risk example also illustrates how you can "pretend" that odds ratios and RR are the same: 0.005 baseline $\times$ 4.75 RR = 0.024, or 2.4%.
>
> However, if the baseline risk for this cancer were 8% and the odds ratio remained 4.75, you must convert the 8% to odds $(0.08 \div 0.92 = 0.09)$, multiply the product by the odds ratio $(4.75 \times 0.09 = 0.43)$, and then reconvert the answer to probability $(0.43 \div 1.43 = 0.3 = 30\%)$. If you treated the odds ratio as an RR in this case, you would have obtained 38%, not 30%; the discrepancy in the use of the two concepts becomes more apparent. Once again, odds are the only choice as the baseline risk rises much above 1%.

Note that baseline risk data cannot be derived from a case-control study because the methodology does not generate prevalence data for the risk factor, so this data must be obtained elsewhere. The typical sequence is that observational suspicion of risk leads to the development of a case-control study; when this study confirms the association, cross-sectional studies are performed to define the prevalence of the risk. Ideally a prospective cohort study then confirms the observation.

One cautionary point to note is that case-control studies are inherently lower in "inference power" than cohort studies. Thus use of odds ratios derived from case-control studies to predict postexposure risk, although mathematically sound, is not encouraged other than for purposes of broad generalization.

## Weighing Risk Avoidance against Disease Prevention

This discussion has covered the use of evidence to estimate a patient's disease likelihood both with and without exposure to the risk factor. The consequences of risk exposure clearly have both a frequency and an impact, the latter of which is highly personal and variable for each patient. This factor is entirely analogous to the issues involved in treatment decisions. Thus construction of an action threshold (AT) for risk decisions is feasible; the process is the same as that involved in treatment decisions and can be best thought of as a threshold analysis for *risk avoidance*—the point at which the benefits of being risk free outweigh the cost and effort necessary to avoid the risk. Readers should recall the original formula for the determination of the AT is as follows:

$$AT = \frac{\text{harm (impact} \times \text{frequency)}}{\text{improvement (impact} \times \text{frequency)}}$$

In risk decisions the harm component becomes the risk-avoidance measures, and the improvement becomes the reduction in disease. Because risk-avoidance measures apply to all patients considering the decision, its frequency is always 1. The AT formula modified for use in risk decisions is as follows:

$$AT_{Risk} = \frac{\text{risk avoidance (impact} \times 1)}{\text{improvement (impact} \times \text{ARR)}}$$

or

$$AT_{Risk} = \frac{\text{risk avoidance impact}}{\text{improvement impact} \times \text{ARR}}$$

Consider the following examples demonstrating such use of the AT.

| *Example* |

Your patient has developed moderate allergic rhinitis symptoms after buying a cat 2 years previous, despite optimal treatment including desensitization. The cat has become the center of her existence, providing great emotional support and enjoyment. An allergy evaluation demonstrates a high likelihood that the symptoms are related to cat dander and thus have a 90% chance of resolving if the cat is removed from the environment.

For this patient the impact of giving away the cat (risk avoidance) is considerable, and she estimates it at 0.3. The allergy symptoms and their required treatments have an impact for her of 0.2. The AT is as follows:

$$AT_{Risk} = \frac{0.3}{0.9 \times 0.2} = 1.7$$

Any value greater than 1 makes the avoidance measures inappropriate for this patient. The patient should keep the cat. In this example the patient likely would not require a quantitative decision analysis but would state a preference at once. In other words the patient would "know" intuitively that the impact of losing her furry companion would be greater than the annoyance of chronic rhinitis. Readers are advised to repeat this scenario, using as a patient a less ardent cat-lover who assesses the removal of the cat with an impact of 0.1 rather than 0.3.

**Example**

In a large epidemiologic cohort study the risk of clinical coronary disease in healthy, middle-aged men at average risk was around 10% over 10 years.[3] Assume that moderate exercise decreased this risk to 6% (for a 4% AR reduction over 10 years).

Now examine this scenario quantitatively. The impact of the risk avoidance behavior (exercise) can vary enormously. On the one hand a patient who actually enjoys exercise has no decision at all because the avoidance measure is enjoyable and the improvement in risk is greater than 0. Exercising is the only rational decision.

On the other hand, some patients consider exercise so unpleasant as to affect their quality of life negatively, with a value of 0.02, for instance, on a scale of 0 to 1. If the impact of a coronary disease (for example, an equal chance of angina, heart attack, or death) is high (for example, 0.9 in aggregate) and its reduction in frequency over 10 years is 0.04 (that is, 4%), the equation might appear as follows:

$$AT_{Risk} = \frac{\text{risk avoidance impact}}{\text{improvement impact} \times \text{ARR}}$$

$$AT_{Risk} = \frac{0.02}{0.9 \times 0.04} = 0.55$$

Even by the patient's own value system the trouble of exercise appears well worth the effort over a 10-year period because the AT for risk is less than 1. In fact, at some point between 5 and 6 years, the hassle actually provides beneficial results.

**Practical Considerations** Rarely does a practitioner analyze lifestyle risks as quantitatively as in the previous examples. However, these scenarios provide interesting insights into how practitioners can present information to their patients. For example, consider the following creative approach that the previous analysis might support.

> ### Example
>
> You may make the following statement to a patient who you know does not enjoy exercise but who you believe may benefit by reduced risk of heart disease:
>
> "Bill, I know you do not like to exercise. Although we can find ways to minimize its inconvenience and unpleasantness, I suspect we will never make it enjoyable for you. But I want you to consider this: based on your feelings about having heart trouble, we can estimate that it would take only about 5 years of exercise for the benefits to outweigh the hassles. In other words, if you had only 5 years left to live, the trouble of exercise might not be worth the benefit. However, your life expectancy is far greater than that, so the inconvenience of exercising will produce big payoffs in terms of avoiding heart problems down the road. It's an investment that would break even after 5 years and profit indefinitely thereafter."

The sample approach used in the previous scenario can provide the physician with a solid feeling about whether to recommend risk-avoidance measures. Unfortunately, most such recommendations involve risk avoidance, which entails the changing of an unhealthy lifestyle. The reasons for widespread noncompliance in such matters clearly lie beyond the realm of decision analysis.

## SUMMARY

This chapter has focused on risk factors unassociated with the known harm of treatment. These factors include lifestyle and environmental exposures. Although occasional RCTs or cohort studies can be found regarding risks, other types of risk can be studied with case-control methodology only. Parameters often used include the AR (and its inverse, NNH) and RR, both for cohort studies, as well as the newly presented odds ratio (for case-control studies).

Assessing the validity of a case-control study can be difficult. Odds ratios are derived from case-control studies that, although vulnerable to several types of bias and validity concerns, are often the only feasible study method. The physician's task in patient care is to decide whether the risk justifies the patient's making lifestyle or other changes to reduce the likelihood of the undesirable outcome. This decision analysis can be accomplished by comparison of the impact of risk avoidance measures on the one hand against the likelihood and impact of the risk consequences on the other.

# REFERENCES

1. Axelson O and others: Use of the prevalence ratio v the prevalence odds ratio as a measure of risk in cross sectional studies, *Occup Environ Med* 51(8):574, 1994.
2. Fletcher RH and others: *Clinical epidemiology: the essentials,* ed 3, Baltimore, 1996, Williams & Wilkins.
3. Haapanen N and others: Association of leisure time physical activity with the risk of coronary heart disease, hypertension and diabetes in middle-aged men and women, *Int J Epidemiol* 26(4):739-747, 1997.
4. Haynes RB and others: Developing optimal search strategies for detecting clinically sound studies in Medline, *J M Med Inform Assoc* 1:447-458, 1994.
5. Williams BC: Odds ratio and relative risk, *Ann Intern Med* 111(5):444-445, 1989.
6. Zhang J, Yu KF: What's the relative risk? A method of correcting the odds ratio in cohort studies of common outcomes, *JAMA* 280(19):1690-1691, 1998.

# CHAPTER 6

# *Prognosis*

## INTRODUCTION

Prognosis information is a high priority for patients with nontrivial diseases. In social conversation, one of the questions concerned family and friends first ask when they are faced with an unfamiliar diagnosis is: "What's the prognosis?"

Readers should recognize that the question is essentially subjective in that it seeks a reply such as *good* or *serious*. As a practitioner of evidence-based decision making (EBDM), the physician must consider both the subjective component of prognosis and the more objective, quantitative components.

### Impacts

Whereas impacts carry great importance in the decision calculations for diagnosis and treatment decisions, in decisions involving prognosis they are important less for purposes of calculation than as a means to acknowledge the relative priority of an outcome for the patient. Physicians do not often assign numeric values to the impacts of the outcomes that comprise a disease's prognosis but often may be struck by the ways in which different patients might react to the "same" prognosis.

| Example |
| --- |

On considering extensive surgery for a cancer of the jaw, an older patient with a close family is informed that surgery has a high likelihood of leaving him with a visible deformity but also that cure is likely. The patient is relieved that the cancer can be cured and, although not pleased with the prospect of a cosmetic deformity, he pays it little heed.

Faced with the same prognosis, a younger patient in an active social circle is crushed emotionally. She knows she must proceed to achieve a cure but is devastated by the prospect of a cosmetic deformity.

Is the disease prognosis the same for these two patients? Statistically it is. Humanistically, the discrepancy is clear. The numeric parameters of prognosis do not address this issue explicitly, but readers are urged to remain aware of the impact of the outcomes for the patient at hand; the numbers alone do not tell the full story for any patient.

In the purest sense, prognosis consists of an inventory of anticipated outcomes, along with their respective likelihoods and timing. The subjective issues discussed previously form the spiritual or value-based canvas on which these quantities are drawn.

# *Components of Prognosis Decisions*

## UNDERSTANDING THE NUMERIC PARAMETERS OF PROGNOSIS

### Likelihood

The numeric representation of a disease's prognosis consists of the likelihood of each important disease outcome. The physician should tailor this prognosis to whether treatment is anticipated because most diseases behave differently with treatment than without it. In a very real sense the physician already will have discussed prognosis in addressing whether to proceed with treatment at all (the likelihood of certain outcomes without treatment compared with those likelihoods with treatment). For purposes of this discussion, *prognosis* refers to the prognosis of a disease after a treatment decision has been made.

### Timing

Patients benefit from knowing when an outcome can be expected. The prospect of death within a few weeks clearly is different from that of death within a few years. In fact, explaining as clearly as possible how an outcome tends to distribute itself over time is an important task. For example, examine two diseases, both of which are 100% fatal within 2 years; these diseases are portrayed graphically in Figure 6.1.

An accurate statement about both patterns of survival is that the disease is virtually always fatal within 2 years. However, the two graphs portray prognoses that are quite different from each other. In Figure 6.1, *A,* almost all patients sur-

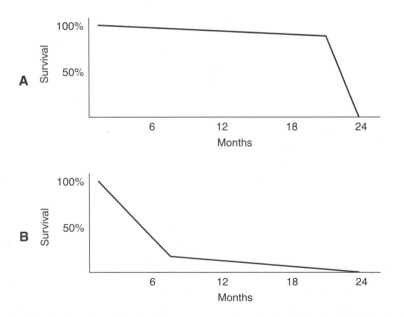

**Figure 6.1**    Both graphs describe a disease with a 2-year mortality of 100%. **A,** Nearly all individuals with this disease survive approximately 20 months. **B,** The majority of individuals with this disease die within the first 8 months or so.

vive for 20 months or so, with heavy mortality concentrated in the last 4 months. A patient who requires 1½ years to achieve certain life milestones and meet various life-planning needs could be assured fairly confidently that the time span is realistic. By contrast, Figure 6.1, *B*, depicts a heavy mortality in the first 8 months; the few survivors gradually die over the subsequent 16 months. A patient faced with this prognosis would be well advised to attend to important planning issues promptly; although hope remains for continued survival up to 2 years, to count on this time span for life-planning purposes would not be prudent.

Another frequently used parameter for prognosis is median survival (or median time until the outcome in question occurs). This time is that in which half the patients will experience the outcome. Again, this "event" may occur all at once or gradually; thus this number alone does not reflect the whole picture a patient needs to fully understand the prognosis.

Timing is not a simple matter. Depending on how the physician describes the two scenarios presented previously, the patient may glean a number of significantly different images. Prognostic information thus should be complete enough to elucidate such timing trends for the patient.

Often the case, especially with mortality, is that the only way to communicate the prognosis accurately and comprehensively to a patient is to use graphs or "word pictures" similar to those displayed in Figure 6.1. When the patient asks, "How long do I have?" a physician's response may be to draw a graph or to reply in a manner that portrays the full time span accurately, as follows:

> *"About half the patients we treat for this disease survive for 1 year. Of those who do, many continue to live for several more years, although by 5 years, only a few patients have survived."*

> *"The vast majority of patients survive in reasonably good health for a year or two. After that, about half survive another year, with only a few surviving beyond the third year."*

In any case the physician may find that the addition of a qualifying statement is both accurate and reassuring to the patient. For instance, the physician may want to stress that this information is statistical in nature, that some patients fare much better than the average, and that medical advances that might change the prognosis may occur at any time.

# *Evidence about Prognosis*

# UNDERSTANDING CLINICAL STUDIES ABOUT PROGNOSIS

## General Considerations

Clinical studies of prognosis generally take the form of cohort studies. A group of individuals with a disease is identified, with a clear and well-accepted diagnosis established by the gold standard, if possible, and with an explicit delineation of the diagnostic criteria being used.

If possible, the cohort should include patients at a comparable stage of the disease. Depending on the researchers' particular interest, this point in the evolution of the disease may be any point in its course, but it should be uniform for the cohort at large. Typically the earlier stages of disease are more productive to study because they eventually will include prognostic information for later stages as the disease progresses.

Such a population generally must be compared with a baseline of similar individuals who do not have the disease to determine how often the outcomes *would have* occurred in an otherwise comparable population. Some studies rely on various actuarial life tables (particularly those focusing on morbidity) that correct for age, race, gender, and similar demographic reference data. If the physician has reason to believe that the diseased cohort does not represent its healthy counterparts in the general population, the accuracy of the evidence should be questioned.

The term *adjusted* often is used to describe the prognosis (or risk) of a disease after correction for the outcomes that would have been expected in a nondiseased population. In 90-year-old individuals with chronic leukemia, for instance, the mortality over the next 5 years may be very high. However, the mortality for age-matched controls (90-year-olds without leukemia) is also "high" relative to younger individuals. In an examination of the prognosis of the leukemia, the expected mortality should be adjusted so that the "excess" mortality from the disease itself can be ascertained.

Another potential confounder is that in most populations with serious illness, patients receive treatment. Withholding treatment known to be effective is clearly unethical, and patients who decline such treatment may not represent the group at large. Thus practitioners seeking cohort studies should be alert to whether the study is one of treated patients, untreated patients, or both. As opposed to treatment studies that assign subjects randomly and prospectively to receive treatment or not, prognosis cohort studies must control for this factor statistically.

Assessing the course of a disease can be subject to bias if the investigators know about certain individual factors they believe affect outcomes; that is, if one researcher believes that subjects who smoke will fare worse than those who do not, the investigator may be inclined subconsciously to detect clinical symptoms and signs more readily in smokers than in nonsmokers. For this reason, to the extent that the parameters being followed have a subjective component to their interpretation or identification, the researchers should be "blind" to the subjects' status to the greatest extent possible. In most studies the outcomes being studied are fairly objective, but as always the practitioner seeking evidence should be especially alert when one or more outcomes are open to subjective judgment; these situations are those in which blinding is a valuable criterion.

## Subgroup Analysis

Every large cohort can be subdivided into smaller component groups. Important information can be gleaned if such subgroup analysis is performed carefully. For example, a study of multiple sclerosis showed that subjects with initially unremitting and progressive disease fared worse than those with relapsing disease.[5] Similarly, certain age or clinical subgroups often have different prognoses.

The caution about this type of analysis is that in virtually any large enough study, patterns that portend especially good or bad prognoses due to chance alone can be identified *retrospectively.* This situation is a bit like the finding of prophesy in the phone book with a search for every 16th or 19th or 27th word on pages 389 through 413, for instance; looking hard enough with enough creative thinking can produce almost any association. Furthermore, a subgroup selected for one conspicuous trait (for example, age or lifestyle) feasibly may be at risk for a different prognosis from the group as a whole not because of the selected trait, but rather for some *other* associated trait that has not been identified.

The practitioner's best assurance when encountering such a finding from a subgroup analysis is to ascertain whether the tested hypothesis was considered *before* the study results were known *(a priori)* and, even more accurately, whether the finding was validated with a separate (usually smaller) study. For this validation the investigators would identify an independent population (not derived from the original study population) having the subgroup profile identified in the original study; this population would be followed prospectively to determine whether the subjects followed the course predicted by their subgroup risk profile.

*Example*

A hypothetic study was designed to determine whether caffeine use decreased survival rates of individuals with pancreatic cancer. After extensive statistical analysis, the researchers determined that no valid association existed between the two factors. However, an astute investigator noticed a curious trend suggesting that subjects who used Styrofoam cups rather than ceramic cups seemed to experience a greater mortality. The researchers performed further analysis to investigate Styrofoam-cup users specifically. Indeed a small but statistically significant increase in mortality existed in this subgroup.

Given only the information provided in the example, the astute reader would greet with great skepticism the apparent cause-and-effect association between Styrofoam-cup use and pancreatic cancer. On the other hand, had the investigators tested their hypothesis by assembling a new, independent group of Styrofoam-cup users and followed those subjects in a cohort study, comparing them against the general similar population, a much more convincing argument could be made in favor of the hypothesis.

### How Long to Watch

The duration of prognosis studies of chronic disease is a source of potential concern. If the period of study is too short, the full nature of the disease course remains unseen; if it is too long, the inevitable dropout rate mounts, and the reader must make assumptions about the fate of those subjects. When the dropout number grows large, the validity of the study diminishes. Researchers and readers of such studies may need to apply considerable medical and biologic knowledge to determine how long the study "should" be.

## RETRIEVING EVIDENCE ABOUT PROGNOSIS

### The Master Prognosis Evidence Question

The Master Prognosis Evidence Question is as follows:

> *What are the likelihoods and time distributions of the anticipated disease outcomes?*

At least three issues must be addressed in situations involving prognosis, as follows:

1. **Impact**—the subjective importance of each outcome for the individual patient
2. **Outcomes**—the characterization of all important outcomes of interest and their likelihoods
3. **Timing**—the time frames of the important outcomes, including when they occur and how long they last

Preappraised data repositories may provide time savings and filtering for high-quality research. When these databases fail to meet the evidence needs, however, the practitioner should turn to MEDLINE.

Prognosis evidence has its own two-pass search strategy, just as other categories of evidence feature specific search strategies. The following strategy is recommended:

**Pass 1:** index terms AND (incidence OR prognos*)
**Pass 2:** #1 AND (cohort* OR follow-up)

Example

An active patient has developed "tennis elbow," which has responded to conservative measures but seems to recur regularly. She asks you whether the condition likely will progress so that she can decide whether to continue playing tennis or switch to another recreational activity.

**Pass 1:** epicondylitis AND (incidence OR prognosis)
*Results:* 177

**Pass 2:** #1 AND (cohort* OR follow-up)
*Results:* 17

The 177 articles found under pass 1 contain very few applicable to the question at hand. Of peripheral interest is one article about treatment, showing that although local steroid injections resulted short-term relief of symptoms, by 1 year about 84% of subjects in both the injection group and the control group demonstrated significant improvement.[3] Although this study was a randomized controlled trial (RCT) of treatment, it does illustrate that prognostic information often can be obtained by a review of the outcomes of the placebo group in a therapy study.

The final 17 articles included one with a systematic overview of available evidence on the prognosis of tennis elbow.[4] It concluded that the methodologic quality of available studies is low, that long-term studies are particularly lacking, and that prior occurrences of the disease suggest a poorer prognosis.

The tennis elbow example illustrates a common occurrence in real-world medical practice. Despite use of optimal search methods, the user finds a "hodgepodge" of evidence but no definitive evidence. Still, a fair amount of information can be gleaned from the previous search results. For example, if one study shows a 15% persistence rate for symptoms at 1 year and a second study suggests that patients with previous occurrences of this disease have worse prognoses than those without prior occurrence, a reasonable step may be for the physician to counsel the patient that the best available research demonstrates that at 1 year a 15% or greater persistence of pain may occur. This statement does not tell the patient whether to continue playing tennis, but it does provide some useful information the patient can use to make a decision.

---

**Example**

A woman experiences a deep vein thrombosis (DVT) in her 20s, at which time she is told she has a familial clotting tendency called *factor V Leiden mutation.* She wonders what the likelihood of a recurrence would be if she became pregnant.

**Pass 1:** deep vein thrombosis AND pregnancy AND factor V Leiden AND (incidence OR prognos*)
*Results:* 19

**Pass 2:** #1 AND (cohort* OR follow-up)
*Results:* 4

Among the four articles found under pass 2, one retrospective study demonstrated an incidence of 0.71 cases of DVT per 1000 deliveries in a general population. In addition, 80% of DVT patients underwent subsequent evaluation for factor V Leiden mutation, 8% of whom tested positive. Based on this very small number, a statistic analysis concluded that the risk of DVT during pregnancy in the presence of factor V Leiden mutation is approximately 1:400.[8] Based on the retrospective nature of the study, the broad confidence intervals surrounding the data, and the lack of explicit diagnostic criteria, a practitioner should be reluctant to rely on these numbers.

Another study focused only on the prevalence of the mutation in pregnant females who had a thrombosis,[2] not relevant to the DVT example. A look back at the results of pass 1 reveal that the number of finds is manageable. One cross-sectional study demonstrated an incidence of thrombosis during pregnancy of 28% in factor V Leiden carriers, compared with "under 1%" in unaffected individuals.[1] The practitioner, however, concludes that this evidence cannot be used because it is not a prospective or even a case-control study. Entirely possible is that the factor V Leiden mutation group was followed with serial Doppler studies, whereas those without the mutation underwent routine clinical follow-up. In summary, the numbers are not to be trusted.

This detailed example illustrates that ideal prognostic evidence may be difficult to obtain and that extrapolations about prognosis should not be made from retrospective observational data alone.

## JUDGING THE SUITABILITY OF PROGNOSIS EVIDENCE

The guidelines presented in this section draw largely on the original work by the AMA Evidence-Based Medicine Working Group,[6] modified to reflect my own experience in teaching and using this material. These guidelines also are summarized nicely in Sackett's recent text.[9]

### Assessing Applicability

The issues surrounding applicability of evidence about prognosis resemble those pertaining to other types of evidence. Thus the questions the physician must ask to determine applicability are similar to those used with other types of evidence.

### Are the Study Participants Like My Patient?
As with previously discussed types of evidence, the practitioner should look at the age, gender, and other demographic factors that potentially could affect the course of the disease in question. Furthermore, ensuring that the stage of disease represented in the study population includes a substantial representation of patients with the same stage of disease present in the patient in question also is important. Careful dissection of the appropriate numbers from the study may be necessary to determine which numbers actually apply

to the patient at hand, but sufficient representation should exist to reassure the practitioner that the results are indeed applicable.

In clinical situations, extenuating circumstances often may be present that are unique to the individual patient. Normally, finding evidence that is specific to the patient at hand is difficult or impossible. In such cases the practitioner may find it useful to derive the prognostic information as though the unique circumstances were not present, use these data as an anchor point, and modify the data accordingly to account for the unique circumstances. This approach at least provides a sensible baseline from which to start, rather than forcing the practitioner to discard the available evidence altogether.

### Are All the Important Prognostic Factors Considered?

Although most studies pay careful attention to the significant prognostic factors, the individual patient may be especially concerned about specific outcomes not addressed by the research. Common sense dictates that all factors important to that patient be addressed. The situation in which this dilemma occurs most frequently in my experience is that of serious illnesses. Evidence may be retrieved that addresses mortality and major complications, but lesser complications that are nonetheless important for quality-of-life considerations may not be addressed explicitly in the relevant research.

In situations in which two or more additional factors may affect prognosis, aside from the main factor under study, the practitioner should ensure that the study's researchers adjusted for these considerations in their final analysis. Adjusted odds ratios and hazard ratios are common parameters used to report such adjustments.

## Assessing Validity

The practitioner also must consider certain criteria when assessing a study's validity.

### Is the Cohort Described Well and Generally at a Consistent Stage in the Progression of the Disease?

The study should provide sufficient information about the population for the practitioner to determine whether it truly represents the population the authors state they are studying. For example, if an article claims to describe the general prognosis of rheumatoid arthritis, it should reveal how that population was assembled. If the subjects all were selected from a tertiary referral center, they may not represent the patients a primary-care physician is likely to encounter in private practice. The prognosis for one population may not be the same as that for another.

Ensuring that the stage of disease within the population is reasonably uniform also is important. If a mixture of individuals with early- and late-stage disease exist, the practitioner may be unable to use the study's evidence to help the patient in question. Ideally the uniform stage of disease would be relatively early in its course.

### Were the Outcomes Measured Objectively and Appraised Comparably for All Participants? If Outcomes Were Open to Subjective Interpretation, Were the Researchers Blinded as to Each Participant's History?

Outcomes with measurements or assessments that have subjective components must be examined carefully. The researcher performing the assessment should be blinded to the participant's disease status and to any other factors that conceivably could create bias.

In addition, all outcomes should be measured identically for all study participants, regardless of disease severity, demographic factors, and any other variables. In the previous example a retrospective design resulted in the possibility that individuals with the disease in question (factor V Leiden mutation) received frequent ultrasound diagnostic tests, whereas individuals without the disease simply were followed clinically. Not surprisingly the prognosis for the disease revealed an exceedingly high incidence of DVT because the disease-group outcomes were measured far differently than the outcomes in the other group.

### Was Follow-Up of the Study Group Performed Thoroughly, and Did the Follow-Up Period Last Long Enough?

These criteria are relatively self-explanatory, although ample clinical judgment is required to determine how long is "long enough" and how thorough is "thorough enough." As with studies of therapy, the practitioner should ensure that the dropout rate is sufficiently small to permit the drawing of a valid conclusion. If it is not, the practitioner may choose to regard the results in the following two ways:

1. As if all the participants who dropped out sustained the outcome of interest
2. As if all the participants who dropped out did *not* develop the outcomes of interest

In this way the practitioner can create both a best-prognosis scenario and a worst-prognosis scenario for the patient.

### Did the Study Account for Important Factors that Might Have Affected Outcomes?

To understand this criterion, consider the prognosis of pneumonia. If the study failed to account for the tobacco usage of participants, its results might be quite misleading. Similarly, the simultaneous presence of diseases such as diabetes, asthma, or immune deficiency would be important incidental prognostic factors for pneumonia. When reviewing prognosis studies, practitioners should consider which factors, aside from the disease in question, might affect the outcomes of interest and determine whether the investigators accounted for these factors in their final results.

In addition, practitioners must remember that validity is a relative quality. Whenever compromises based on failure to adhere to the previously stated cri-

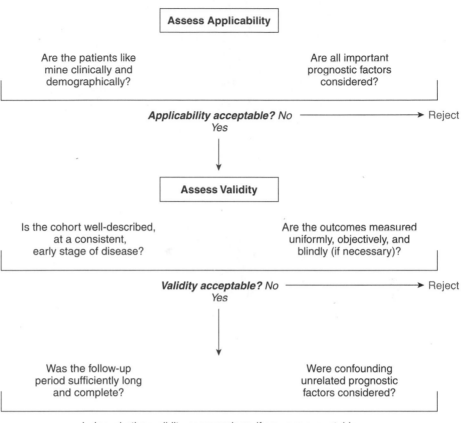

**Figure 6.2**　Summary of appraisal of prognostic evidence. Note that *accept* and *reject* are two extremes of inference as to how closely a study approximates the "truth." Most physicians' interpretations generally fall somewhere between the two extremes.

teria are present, the judgment of the practitioner ultimately determines whether these compromises render the evidence unusable for the patient at hand. In other words, threats to a study's validity are often not black or white, but rather shades of gray. The practitioner's judgment may be the final determinant of whether to accept or reject the conclusions of the study.

Figure 6.2 summarizes the appraisal process for evidence about prognosis.

# *Helping the Patient Decide*

# USING PROGNOSIS EVIDENCE IN MEDICAL DECISIONS

## The Master Decision Question

The Master Decision Question in matters of prognosis is as follows:

*Does awareness of the likelihoods of the various outcomes over time help my patient make important life decisions?*

Imagining a scenario in which a patient would be better served not knowing the prognosis of a disease is difficult. A practical question is to decide just how precisely and with what degree of confidence the prognosis should be delineated quantitatively. For patients suffering from upper-respiratory infections a simple "you should be much better in a few days" often is sufficient. On the other hand, a patient faced with a potentially fatal malignancy may desire a much more exacting response.

The question of whether a prognosis (or an individual outcome) is considered "good" or "bad" is highly subjective. Certainly, scenarios exist at each end of the spectrum about which most observers would agree. On the other hand, a patient's personal priorities and values may affect how that individual feels about the likelihood of a given outcome at a certain point in time.

Given the previous statements, the difficulty involved in speaking in general terms about the use of prognostic evidence in medical decision making is understandable. Rather, such evidence applies primarily to *personal* decision making, such as life-events planning, financial and legal steps, and emotional and spiritual preparation for death or disability. In the case of very serious diseases, prognostic evidence also allows for appropriate planning of palliative care or hospice arrangements.

Once the physician has educated the patient in a general way about a serious disease, inquiring about how the potential disease outcomes will affect that patient is crucial. The answers do not change the prognosis, but they do help the physician focus counseling on those issues the patient considers important. For instance, does an elderly, celibate patient care about the likelihood of sexual dysfunction as much as a younger, sexually active individual? Does a fatal outcome in several years have the same importance to a patient with an unrelated terminal illness as it does to a healthy patient?

In general, the prognostic evidence most useful to the patient is that evidence affecting the patient's choices about life planning, treatment, and emotional adjustments. The physician's obligation is to ensure that the information is accurate and free of distortion.

## Helping Patients Interpret Prognostic Numbers

**Medians and Probabilities** The prognostic information for amyotrophic lateral sclerosis (Lou Gehrig disease) has been summarized as shown in Table 6.1.[7,10] Although certain prognostic factors were identified that alter these figures, this example focuses on the numbers only.

## TABLE 6.1

**Prognostic Information Relating to Amyotrophic Lateral Sclerosis Patients**

|  | A. Years from Diagnosis | |
|---|---|---|
|  | 3 | 5 |
| Likelihood of survival | 29% | 4% |
|  | B. Disease Form | |
|  | Spinal | Bulbar |
| Median survival | 26 months | 12.1 months |

Data from Lee JR and others: Prognosis of amyotrophic lateral sclerosis and the effect of referral selection, *J Neurol Sci* 132(2):207-215, 1995; and Tysnes OB and others: Prognostic factors and survival in amyotrophic lateral sclerosis, *Neuroepidemiology* 13(5):226-235, 1994.

Which of these two forms of presenting data is more useful to the patient? In Table 6.1, *A*, the natural focus is on the likelihood (probability) of death at a specific point in time. This information is not well suited to help the patient answer the question, "How long do I have to live?" Although the patient can surmise from this information that the likelihood of surviving even 3 years is quite low, many patients would conclude from this data little more than an impression of having 3 years or less to live.

Conversely, Table 6.1, *B*, may provide more useful information. A patient with the spinal form of this disease has an "even chance" of surviving 26 months; therefore this figure serves as an "anchor point" for how long the patient might expect to live, given at least average "luck." This figure provides a median—the time at which half of all patients would have succumbed and half would have survived.

### Example

A patient with a newly diagnosed incurable cancer poses the question, "What is the prognosis?" As a sensitive EBDM practitioner, you pause before answering this question directly. Instead, you respond to the patient's needs by separating the various elements possibly implied by the term *prognosis*. Thus you choose not to reply initially with a statement such as the following:

*"Approximately 60% of patients will survive 4 years, and 10% will survive 5 years."*

Instead, you might respond with the following sort of answer:

*"At least half of all patients with this disease survive 4 years. Quite a few survive much longer. The vast majority of patients maintain a very high quality of life until shortly before they die."*

The second response to the patient's request for a prognosis provides an anchor point for the patient (4 years), a valid expression of hopefulness, and an acknowledgment of the importance of quality of life in addition to survival. Depending on the patient's response to this reply, a skilled physician could provide much more information. By contrast, the first reply in the example appears inadequate and abrupt. Even patients who are mathematically unsophisticated can recognize that this figure (4 years) is not a precise predictor, but many are likely to find significant information contained in the numbers provided.

**Interpreting the Timing of Events** An earlier discussion in the chapter examined how two scenarios can appear similar if described in one fashion and quite different if described in another. Consider the following example.

Example

Two diseases share a 2-year mortality rate of 100%. The first disease has essentially a 4%-per-month mortality. The second has almost no mortality in the first 20 months but a very severe, virtually universal mortality in the last 4 months.

An important point for the patient who encounters such a disease is that the physician examine not only the "bottom line" event rate when interpreting prognostic evidence but also the dynamics with which that event occurs. Cohort studies generally provide such detail, but only through knowing the patient can physicians determine which figures are most important to them.

Notwithstanding the difficulty in generalizations about how to use prognostic information in medical decision making, one factor that is consistently important is to provide the information *in a way that most directly answers the question the patient is asking*.

The interpersonal dynamics of presenting prognostic information are beyond the scope of this book. However, readers should understand clearly that the way in which prognostic evidence is reported to the patient can have a major impact on the physician's ability to respond to the patient's needs.

## SUMMARY

This chapter has examined how the concept of prognosis implies both the likelihood of certain outcomes, as well as their impact on the patient's life. Such evidence can be presented in numerous ways, and selection of the format that best addresses the questions the patient addresses is important.

Generally the strongest evidence about prognosis comes from cohort studies. Descriptive studies are common, but they should be viewed as anecdotal and hypothesis-raising, rather than as evidence. Searching for evidence about prognosis can be done in a two-pass method using specific syntax. The suitability of prognostic evidence depends on the assessment of its applicability (adequate representation of the patient in question in the study population both demographically and clinically) and validity (a well-defined population with sufficient follow-up and objective measurement of outcomes).

Patients' use of prognostic evidence is a highly personal matter, affecting life-planning issues ranging from momentous when the disease is serious to routine when the disease is of less consequence (for example "When can I count on going back to work?"). The physician must present the evidence to patients in a manner consistent with the way in which that patient is likely to use it.

## REFERENCES

1. Dizon-Townson DS and others: The incidence of the factor V Leiden mutation in an obstetric population and its relationship to deep vein thrombosis, *Am J Obstet Gynecol* 176(4):883-886, 1997.
2. Hallak M and others: Activated protein C resistance (factor V Leiden) associated with thrombosis in pregnancy, *Am J Obstet Gynecol* 176(4):889-893, 1997.
3. Hay EM and others: Pragmatic randomised controlled trial of local corticosteroid injection and naproxen for treatment of lateral epicondylitis of elbow in primary care, *BMJ* 319 (7215):964-968, 1999.
4. Hudak PL and others: Understanding prognosis to improve rehabilitation: the example of lateral elbow pain, *Arch Phys Med Rehabil* 77(6):586-593, 1996.
5. Kremenchutzky M and others: The natural history of multiple sclerosis: a geographically based study. 7. Progressive-relapsing and relapsing-progressive multiple sclerosis: a re-evaluation, *Brain* 122(Pt 10):1941-1950, 1999.
6. Luapacis A and others, for the Evidence-Based Medicine Working Group: Users' guides to the medical literature. V. How to use an article on prognosis, *JAMA* 272:234-237, 1994.
7. Lee JR and others: Prognosis of amyotrophic lateral sclerosis and the effect of referral selection, *J Neurol Sci* 132(2):207-215, 1995.
8. McColl MD and others: Risk factors for pregnancy associated venous thromboembolism, *Thromb Haemost* 78(4):1183-1188, 1997.
9. Sackett DL and others: *Evidence-based medicine: how to practice and teach EBM,* ed 2, New York, 2000, Churchill Livingstone.
10. Tysnes OB and others: Prognostic factors and survival in amyotrophic lateral sclerosis, *Neuroepidemiology* 13(5):226-235, 1994.

# CHAPTER 7

# *Evidence Overviews*

## INTRODUCTION

Almost any broad review of a medical topic can present itself as an *overview* or a *review*. This chapter focuses on the systematic review and one of its subtypes, known as the *meta-analysis*.

In any perusal of the literature, *review articles* appear frequently on timely topics. These should not be confused with those known as *systematic reviews*. Review articles typically are updated discussions of a clinical topic by authors who are experienced in the area. They may appear in distinguished, peer-reviewed journals and in less rigorously reviewed publications. When such articles are written with due attention to the current evidence, they are excellent sources of up-to-date background knowledge and provide convenient references to evidence reports. If a phrase such as *state-of-the-art* appears in the title, the work is likely a review article. In less-discerning examples, review articles detail the experience and style of an author, providing little support from the primary literature, and are filled with recommendations and colorful "pathways" that may make for interesting reading but are not reliable sources for use in evidence-based medicine (EBM).

Regardless of the quality of a review article of this type, the work should not be considered true *evidence*. It may help the physician retrieve good evidence, and that physician may rely on it for clinical management, but such articles always are essentially sources of background knowledge.

Systematic reviews, discussed in the following section, provide a more focused type of article designed to summarize the current state of the evidence about a specific clinical question.

# Components of Systematic Reviews

# UNDERSTANDING SYSTEMATIC REVIEWS

## Standard Systematic Reviews

The term *systematic review (SR)* refers to a formal and usually exhaustive review of the evidence pertaining to a focused topic. When done rigorously, such a review can save the practitioner a great deal of effort. Furthermore, it is presented in such a way that practitioners can gauge the quality of the evidence and quickly glean the core numbers that may prove necessary. The methodology used to retrieve and appraise the evidence is described explicitly so that the practitioner can judge whether the authors' standards are adequate for the case at hand. In the best case the conclusions are as close to a definitive statement of evidence as any practitioner can hope to find.

The practitioner should seek the following elements to identify a well-executed SR:

1. The question being studied is focused and potentially answerable through use of quantitative parameters.
2. The strategies used to retrieve the evidence are explicitly stated, sound, and exhaustive. The type of evidence considered acceptable is stated prospectively (for example, randomized controlled trials [RCTs] only).
3. The retrieved evidence is reviewed thoroughly and subjected to critical appraisal criteria comparable to those discussed previously and elsewhere in other definitive EBM sources.[5] The conclusions of such appraisals are presented.
4. The evidence culled from this process is "normalized" so that results presented in various ways can be compared in terms of the magnitude of effect. This criterion is not to say that the data are "pooled" but rather that evidence reported in, for instance, absolute risk reduction (ARR) can be compared with different evidence initially reported as relative risk (RR).
5. Conclusions are drawn based on the previous criteria, which are supported by the findings and can be applied to the patient in question.

Rarely do numerous studies about a single topic follow identical paths. One may have a slightly different patient population; another may use different dosing regimens; a third may follow the subjects for a longer time period. Authors of SRs usually address such discrepancies, and practitioners should seek out convincing evidence that these discrepancies do not detract from the conclusions presented.

SRs do not attempt to pool data from different studies into one larger bank of data (that task being left to a meta-analysis, discussed in the following section). Rather, they look at each valid study separately and use the results as a "vote" about the truth. Furthermore, study size counts; larger studies (assuming they are valid) get more votes than smaller ones. Thus the results of a hypothetic SR might read as follows:

> In our research, 34 RCTs of this agent met the methodologic criteria for our review. Of these, 30 showed a beneficial effect, whereas three showed no effect.

One showed an actual worsening of the disease, although this study was done with twice the conventional dose used in the remaining studies. The three studies that failed to show an effect were in subjects older than age 60. The remainder enrolled subjects from ages 35 through 60.

Note how the results are summarized without their data being combined. Many SRs list their component trials in a table that includes study size, results, and other important data the reader can review. In essence the authors of a high-quality SR have done most of the work that the evidence-based practitioner might otherwise do. All that is left is to apply the evidence to the individual patient; no study can ever perform that task.

As readers might imagine, practitioners are pleased to stumble on an excellent SR. However, they must possess the necessary tools to recognize one.

## Meta-Analyses

A more specialized type of SR is the meta-analysis. When numerous sound studies exist about a topic, "pooling" of the results, as if they all pertain to one large study, is possible. At least two reasons exist for this pooling function, as follows:

1. Smaller studies may provide inconclusive results with large confidence intervals (CIs), even when an effect truly is present; the small size precludes a confident interpretation of the trends. When several such studies are pooled, the results may prove statistically significant even when the individual studies fail to do so.
2. When sound studies provide conflicting results, pooling them together may reconcile the data into a single, conclusive result. The size and magnitude of the effects in each study may be "weighed" against and combined with the others in such a way that the practitioner can generate confident conclusions despite the discrepancies among them.

**Understanding How a Meta-Analysis Can Clarify Evidence** Figure 7.1 is a diagram representing several studies on the efficacy of a treatment for a hypothetic disease. The vertical axis represents an RR for the bad outcome of 1, at which the treatment has no effect. Values to the left of this axis have RRs less than 1 and therefore indicate an effective treatment (risk of bad outcomes less than in the untreated population). The black circles are the "point estimates" or actual results of a given study, and the horizontal lines are the 95% CIs for that study.

Assume that the studies in Figure 7.1 are valid RCTs. Following is a summary of conclusions about each individual study:

A. Results showed efficacy but were not statistically significant (its CI including 1).
B. Results showed efficacy but were not statistically significant (its CI including 1).

C. Results showed efficacy but were not statistically significant (its CI in-
cluding 1).
D. Results showed no efficacy and were statistically significant.
E. Results showed efficacy and were statistically significant.

A systematic overview would state the existence of five acceptable studies; of
these, only two show statistical significance. One shows the treatment as efficacious, and the other does not. Therefore insufficient evidence exists to
demonstrate that the treatment works or does not work. Reading this systematic overview, most readers would remain reluctant to use the treatment.

A more careful look at the graph in Figure 7.1, however, reveals clearly that
most of the studies showed a trend favoring treatment. One of the important
reasons why studies fail to achieve acceptable CIs (and therefore statistical significance) is that they are too small. If the results of all the studies are pooled
and recalculated, the results displayed in the meta-analysis row become more
clear: The treatment is efficacious and has a high level of statistical significance.
In pooling of the data, strict attention must be paid to many details, including
study size, comparability, and reporting units. With appropriate attention the
meta-analysis can reveal truths that individual studies do not elucidate.

Readers might imagine how complex the statistical manipulations must be
to combine results of several studies into one larger "virtual" study. Nonstatis-
ticians are virtually unable to appraise critically the technical aspects of such
analyses. However, a simplified example can help illustrate some aspects of the
meta-analysis.

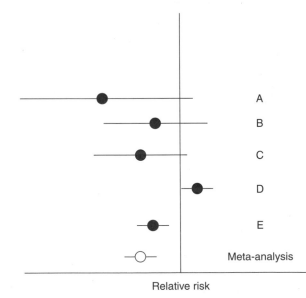

**Figure 7.1**   Five separate studies are represented with their respective 95% confidence intervals *(horizontal lines)*. The vertical axis corresponds to a relative risk of 1, and the black circles indicate the **actual**
results of the studies.

Example

An early study of a drug in the treatment of high blood pressure showed that the drug held a substantial advantage over hydrochlorothiazide, a familiar treatment. Of 30 patients treated, nine (30%) reached a 10% reduction in their systolic pressure readings, whereas of those treated with hydrochlorothiazide, six of 30 (20%) reached that goal. The study was deemed valid and applicable, although the CI around the 10% discrepancy between the two drugs was −12% to 34%. The authors, to their credit, concluded that the difference between the two drugs was not statistically significant.

Then 6 months later a separate group performed a similar study. The researchers noted a 10% blood pressure reduction in 13 of 40 treated patients but in only six of 40 hydrochlorothiazide patients. The difference of 12.5% in the success rate of the two groups had a CI of −1% to 36%. Thus the second study also failed to demonstrate a statistically significant advantage to the new drug. The drug's discoverers were becoming discouraged.

At last, an analyst decided to do a meta-analysis of the topic. She pooled the two previous studies after correcting for minor differences between them. In this case the consolidated "virtual" study demonstrated a 16% discrepancy between the two groups, with a CI of 2% to 30%. Together, with the advantage of a larger pool of patients, the drug was deemed effective and advantageous with statistical significance.

Often I have noticed a reluctance to accept meta-analysis evidence as conclusive evidence, even by experienced practitioners of evidence-based decision making (EBDM). The reasons include unfamiliarity with the techniques of meta-analysis, possible selection bias in the studies the investigators choose to include (unless they include virtually all valid studies available), and the inherent fear of "data-mining," in which data can be manipulated subtly to illustrate any desired result. However, a sound meta-analysis accounts for these pitfalls and often provides the best evidence available on the topic.

A final real-world example is that of a recent study of exercise tests designed to detect coronary disease in women.[3] The positive likelihood ratios for thallium scanning ranged from 1.9 to 6.9 in individual studies, whereas the pooled data showed a result of 2.9 [95% CI 1 to 5]. This pooled figure, along with its marginal statistical significance, reflects the truth far more coherently than the individual studies from which it is drawn.

## RECOGNIZING SYSTEMATIC REVIEWS

Judging the suitability of an SR involves application of the criteria presented in the discussions pertaining to specific categories of evidence. That is, in an SR about a treatment the component studies should be appraised by use of the treatment evidence criteria; likewise in an SR about a diagnostic test, the diagnostic appraisal criteria would be applied.

## Distinguishing Systematic Reviews from Review Articles

Although this discussion has delineated the differences between ordinary review articles and SRs, the distinction is not always obvious in practice. An examination of two overview articles may help illustrate the process by which review articles are distinguished from SRs.

> *Example*

Regarding the treatment of hepatitis B, you find an article entitled, "Chronic hepatitis B virus infection: treatment strategies for the next millennium."[4] The first thing you notice is that the abstract simply reviews certain key points about the disease, without discussing methodology, conclusions, or other topics frequently examined in true SRs.

As you scan the article further, you see that it contains sections similar to those you would expect to see in a textbook, entitled *virologic characteristics, goals of treatment,* and *lamivudine.*

You do not see sections describing search methodology or critical appraisal criteria, nor do you find tabulations of data derived from primary evidence. Therefore you conclude that this work is a review article, as opposed to an SR. Indeed, you find the review article quite useful, with 100 references. Still, you correctly view the article more as an updated textbook chapter than as a source of foreground knowledge.

By contrast, you discover in the same issue of the same journal an article entitled, "A systematic review of newer pharmacologic therapies for depression in adults: evidence report summary."[8] The abstract for this article contains a number of sections—background, purposes, data sources, study selection, data extraction, data synthesis, and conclusions. The article itself contains sections with titles such as *methods, data synthesis, efficacy in children and adolescents,* and *discussion.* Representative excerpts from the methods section read as follows:

*"English-language and non–English-language literature was identified by using the Cochrane Collaboration depression, anxiety and neurosis group's specialized registry of . . ."*

and

*"The terms* depression, depressive disorder, *or* dysthymic disorder *were combined with a list of 32 specific 'newer' and antidepressants . . . to yield 1277 relevant records."*

This article also contains several tables, one summarizing the treatment trials of antidepressants and herbal remedies. Another section specifies that RCTs that lasted at least 6 weeks were required and that clinical outcomes were included in the assessments. Clearly, you determine that this article qualifies as an SR.

## Distinguishing Meta-Analyses from Other Systematic Reviews

Surprisingly, segregation of standard SRs from meta-analyses occasionally can be difficult, especially when the tabular results display counts of studies, means, and other parameters that appear to pool the data.* The clues used to determine a true meta-analysis include the following:

- Individual participant numbers were extracted from each study and re-assessed in a new, aggregated pool of subjects.
- The results for each study were "weighted" to account for the study's size. Terms such as *weighted event rate* and *weighted odds ratios* suggest that this step has been done.
- Tables show individual study sizes plus a row entitled *all studies* or *total*, with full results calculated for the total row.

---

*Individual patient numbers might be tabulated from each study and reassessed as a new, aggregated pool of patients, but unless this action is done in a statistically rigorous way, it does not qualify as a true meta-analysis.

# *Evidence from Systematic Reviews*

## PRESENTATION OF EVIDENCE FROM SYSTEMATIC REVIEWS

The evidence gleaned from SRs reflects the category to which the underlying primary studies belong. Thus a review of a diagnostic test, for example, is likely to provide sensitivity, specificity, or likelihood ratios. Such topics have been discussed in previous chapters.

Because the underlying studies may report their evidence using a variety of parameters, authors of SRs sometimes choose a common denominator when summarizing the aggregate data. In a series of treatment studies, some authors may report absolute risks (ARs) only, whereas others may report RR reductions only. One logical means to introduce consistency into such a collection is to convert all results to RRs (or NNT, odds ratios, or another common unit for all studies) in the final analysis.

In the case of meta-analyses the mathematic requirements are more stringent. In these studies, odds ratios, RRs, and other parameters that may never have been used in the component articles may appear. Use of such common denominators enables the authors to perform quantitative adjustments to the data, allowing them to draw conclusions that might otherwise have gone unrecognized.

## RETRIEVING SYSTEMATIC REVIEWS

The chapter about treatments discussed the Cochrane Library because this source is confined essentially to therapy studies. It is mentioned again in this discussion as one of the richer sources of SRs. Similarly, *ACP Journal Club* and Evidence-Based Medicine, also discussed previously, are repositories of highly appraised reports but are broader in scope because they contain articles of other types as well (for example diagnosis, prognosis, or risk).

In addition, the Health Services/Technology Assessment Text (HSTAT) website (http://text.nlm.nih.gov) is another source of both guidelines and evidence summaries supported by the United States National Library of Medicine. Another promising resource is an Internet-based data center known as *DARE (Database of Abstracts of Reviews of Effectiveness;* http://nhscrd.york. ac.uk/darehp.htm). Supported by the British National Health Service and several health departments in the United Kingdom, the DARE site is maintained at the University of York. DARE is essentially a review of reviews wherein the editors select SRs from MEDLINE and other literature databases. Those authors independently assess the citations and cull the list to those that satisfy explicit inclusion criteria. The final set of reviews then is summarized in an original abstract.

A sample DARE search for the term *sarcoidosis* reveals two reviews—one regarding the use of steroids for treatment and the other about diagnosis via mediastinoscopy. The former was drawn from the Cochrane Database, and detailed summaries are provided for both. By comparison, the Cochrane Database itself was searched for the same term with the Ovid search engine;

five reviews were found, including the one retrieved by DARE. Currently, DARE appears to be a very useful, if incomplete, resource. Because it resembles a hybrid of Best Evidence (in that its breadth includes treatments, risk, diagnosis, and more) and the Cochrane Database (as an explicit, systematized collection of reviews), it has the potential to be a very important initial stop for appraised evidence.

Regarding searching from "scratch" in MEDLINE, my experience is that the first of the two-pass search strategies described in their respective chapters (that is, in the chapter applicable to the type of evidence being sought) reveals most current SRs of interest. Glanville and Lefebvre[2] have suggested the use of a specific filter, reporting a sensitivity of 55% and a precision of 71%. Unfortunately the filter contains 16 separate steps and is thus cumbersome to implement. Although no evidence has been found to suggest a better strategy, a more practical approach might be to search the previously discussed compendia and, if no reviews are found, examine the results of the first pass. I have found useful the implementation of a second filter, as follows:

#1 AND (systematic review OR meta*)

Additional searching beyond this example would rely on an empiric, common sense-based strategy (for example, use of alternative terms in place of the keywords).

## JUDGING THE SUITABILITY OF SYSTEMATIC REVIEWS

### Assessing the Applicability of a Systematic Review

No distinction exists between the applicability of an SR and that of the articles of which it is composed. Thus the lessons learned about applicability for the primary evidence categories can be applied in this discussion as well.

One caveat is to ensure that the spectrum of articles reviewed are consistent in their inclusion of patients. If the patient in question is represented by the subjects in only a few of the many articles reviewed, the results and conclusions of the review may not be a good match. Thus the practitioner has the extra burden not only of checking general applicability issues but also of ensuring that the specific patient descriptors are well represented in the articles of the review.

*Example*

Your patient suffers from osteoarthritis of the knee and is contemplating treatment with acetaminophen. You uncover an SR that focuses on this issue in detail for osteoarthritis in general. Of 17 RCTs reviewed, 15 studied hip arthritis only, whereas two smaller trials focused on knee arthritis. The researchers concluded that acetaminophen was not effective.

In assessing the review's applicability, you correctly note that your patient's disease spectrum was included. However, it was but a small component of the overall meta-analysis. Thus you are not willing to accept the conclusions as applicable. Instead, you perform a more focused search, this time finding a different review that includes only articles about osteoarthritis of the knee.[6] The review concludes that acetaminophen is safe and effective.

## Assessing the Validity of a Systematic Review

Identifying the article as a true SR is only the practitioner's first step in deeming it suitable for the patient at hand. The next step is to determine whether the criteria for validity are met. This chapter does not discuss applicability issues because the concepts discussed in previous chapters would apply equally well to this category. However, validity issues should be considered quite carefully.

### Does This Systematic Review Describe Explicitly Its Search Strategy and the Evidence Resources to Which It Was Applied?

Although the search strategy selected may not be identical to those presented in a textbook such as this, the practitioner should determine whether the strategies appear to be sensitive and reasonably specific. Clues to such a strategy include the use of terms similar to those discussed in this book, medical subject headings (MeSH), and terms that relate to the type of evidence being sought (for example, sensitivity and specificity for diagnostic tests and RCTs for treatments). In addition, the practitioner should include non–English-language research in the search and make an earnest effort to identify "negative" trials, such as those performed through drug company internal research.

### Are the Criteria for Inclusion of a Research Article Clearly Delineated, and Do They Meet Accepted Standards of Critical Appraisal for the Evidence Category in Question?

Standards for evidence discussed in this book provide a suitable background for determination of whether the authors were thoughtful in accepting or discarding a particular study for inclusion in their review. Often, authors use an "evidence-grading system" to help readers judge whether the articles included are of high, average, or low quality. Such a system has been used in various important works, such as the United States Public Health Service (USPHS) report on clinical preventive services.[7] That report contains one of the most careful evidence-rating systems available and has been emulated widely. Table 7.1 summarizes this rating system, whereas Table 7.2 depicts how the authors may use the evidence to arrive at specific recommendations.

The use of terms *good, fair,* and *insufficient* are defined further as they relate to three criteria—the burden of suffering from the condition, the nature of the intervention, and the effectiveness of the intervention based on the reviewed evidence, with an emphasis on the latter element. Thus the recommendation

## Table 7.1
Grades of Evidence

| Grade | Description |
|-------|-------------|
| I | Evidence obtained from at least one properly performed RCT |
| II-1 | Evidence obtained from well-designed controlled trials without randomization |
| II-2 | Evidence obtained from well-designed cohort or case-control analytic studies, preferably from more than one center or research group |
| II-3 | Evidence obtained from multiple time series with or without the intervention; may also encompass dramatic results on uncontrolled experiments (such as the results of the introduction of penicillin treatment in the 1940s) |
| III | Opinions of respected authorities, based on clinical experience; descriptive studies and case reports; or reports of expert committees |

*RCT,* Randomized controlled trial.

## Table 7.2
Grades of Strength of Recommendations

| Grade | Description |
|-------|-------------|
| A | Good evidence to support the recommendation that the condition be considered specifically in a periodic health examination |
| B | Fair evidence to support the recommendation that the condition be considered specifically in a periodic health examination |
| C | Insufficient evidence to recommend for or against the inclusion of the condition in a periodic health examination, but recommendations possible on other grounds |
| D | Fair evidence to support the recommendation that the condition be excluded from consideration in a periodic health examination |
| E | Good evidence to support the recommendation that the condition be excluded from consideration in a periodic health examination |

(decision) process is separated cleanly from the evidence-rating process. This separation is analogous to how the evidence is separated from the decision process throughout this book.

In any appraisal of an SR, the presence of a system such as that used by the USPHS is a good "prognostic factor" for the quality of the work.

### Are the Results of the Review Presented Clearly through Use of Quantitative Parameters Appropriate for the Evidence Category?

The practitioner must judge the quality and consistency of the presentation of quantitative evidence based on the information contained in previous chapters. However, the reality is that some research that was reviewed may have used a system different from what the practitioner expects. Thus the authors

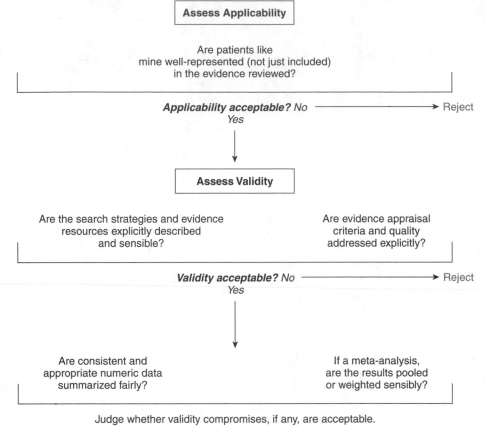

**Figure 7.2** Summary of appraisal of systematic review evidence. Note that *accept* and *reject* are two extremes of inference as to how closely a study approximates the "truth." The average practitioner's interpretation generally falls somewhere between the extremes.

may be obliged to present p-values instead of CIs or other variations of the standard parameters used currently. As long as the quantitative data are presented in a way that the practitioner can understand and compare, the conclusions should be obvious and well supported.

If the answers to the previous three questions concerning validity are acceptable, the SR probably warrants the practitioner's attention. If not, the practitioner might peruse it for valuable information but remain cautious about accepting its conclusions as definitive statements of the "state of the art." Figure 7.2 summarizes the appraisal process for overviews.

# *Helping the Patient Decide*

## USING EVIDENCE BASED ON SYSTEMATIC REVIEWS FOR MEDICAL DECISIONS

The mechanics of decision making from evidence drawn from SRs are those of the underlying evidence categories. Readers are advised to refer to the appropriate chapter for details. However, an important point is to recognize several factors unique to review-derived evidence that might color the decision.

### Strength in Numbers

All other things being equal (if such is ever the case), evidence from SRs is more likely to reflect the truth than is evidence from any single study. For this conclusion to be credible, however, the validity criteria must be followed rigidly. Following are some additional hints that can raise a practitioner's readiness to accept the conclusions as the strongest type of evidence available:

- The collected studies show results that if not almost identical, all align in the same quantitative direction. (For example, they almost all show the treatment to be effective, the RR of a factor to be greater than 1, or the likelihood ratio of a test to be greater than 2.)
- In SRs other than meta-analyses, included studies deemed not statistically significant generally form a trend consistently in the same direction as more conclusive studies. That is, when CIs are too wide (so that they include absolute differences of 0 or RRs of 1), the point estimates are closer to a value suggesting the true effect then they are to the null effect.

> *Example*
>
> Four of eight studies in an SR were deemed not statistically significant because of the following results for RR: 1.2 [95% CI 1.0 to 1.4]; 1.3 [95% CI 0.93 to 1.67]; 0.92 [95% CI 0.8 to 1.4]; and 1.4 [95% CI 0.96 to 1.86]. Although you properly reject the individual findings of these studies because of the lack of statistical significance, if other conclusive studies demonstrated an RR of 1.3, you would be reassured by the fact that of these inconclusive studies, three of four showed a trend toward an average RR in the same direction (greater than 1). This example is a "poor man's" meta-analysis in a sense.

- The authors demonstrate a serious effort to find negative studies to overcome the effect of publication bias. In the case of drug studies this criterion might include the use of manufacturer's internal data, studies reported by personal correspondence to the authors, and attempts to contact recognized experts in the field to determine whether they are aware of other unpublished studies.

### Going Beyond the Evidence

Because SRs acquire the appearance of being "definitive" in nature, the authors may be tempted to make statements in their discussions providing advice about patient management based on their findings. Unfortunately, such statements often fail to meet the same rigorous standards as those the authors applied to their evidence gathering. Ideally, discussion points should be restricted to the final conclusions about the evidence only.

In addition, the factors affecting a patient's decisions are highly unique and personal. Only the physician and the patient can decide whether to implement a plan of care based on the reviewed evidence.

### Example

A rigorous SR of the available evidence reveals that carotid endarterectomy unequivocally improves survival and stroke rates in individuals with greater than 70% occlusion of the internal carotid artery who have experienced recent neurologic symptoms.[1] The study's authors conclude the following:

*"Patients with . . . measured stenosis >70% . . . with a reasonable perioperative risk . . . are likely to benefit from carotid endarterectomy."*

Your patient meets these criteria, and you are about to counsel him accordingly. However, in exploring the issues more carefully, you learn that this patient has two important upcoming milestones—his 50th anniversary in 6 weeks and the birth of a grandson expected in 2 months. Furthermore, he has known locally metastasizing prostate cancer and recently was treated with hormone suppression. Careful reading also reveals that the surgical option carries an RR for death of 2.5 in the 30 days after surgery. Suddenly the unequivocal conclusions of the SR are not so simple.

Your patient decides, with your guidance, that he will wait 3 to 6 months before deciding. By then his personal life will be free of impending milestones and he will know better how his prostate cancer is behaving. Comforted and knowing the risks and benefits, he leaves your office.

SRs, including meta-analyses, should be considered powerful and sophisticated tools used to obtain raw evidence. If the review's authors extend their conclusions to include recommendations for patient management, physicians are advised to scrutinize such well-meaning advice carefully before implementing it for the patient in question.

## SUMMARY

Systematic evidence reviews should be distinguished from ordinary review articles. They provide extraordinary amounts of information and convenience when they are performed rigorously, but they must meet quality criteria similar to those the physician reviewing them would apply in appraising an individual research report. A particularly useful component of an SR is an evidence-rating system. Meta-analyses are a special type of evidence review in which data from independent research are pooled and analyzed as if they were one study.

A sound systematic evidence review reflects the work that an EBM practitioner would perform for the patient; in complex clinical areas that tend to generate the bulk of SRs (for example, hormone replacement for menopause or cholesterol-lowering drugs), the SR provides the most useful type of resource available for EBDM.

Notwithstanding the value of an SR, the actual decision-making process remains individual and subjective. Physicians should use the evidence summary as the raw material for a patient's decision, remembering that the decision is, as always, unique to the individual patient.

## REFERENCES

1. Cina CS and others: Carotid endarterectomy for symptomatic carotid stenosis, *Cochrane Database of Syst Rev* 2:CD001081, 2000.
2. Glanville J, Lefebvre C: Identifying systematic reviews: key resources, *ACP J Club* 132(3):A11-A12, 2000.
3. Kwok Y and others: Meta-analysis of exercise testing to detect coronary artery disease in women, *Am J Cardiol* 83(5):660-666, 1999.
4. Malik AH, Lee WM: Chronic hepatitis B virus infection: treatment strategies for the next millennium, *Ann Intern Med* 132:723-731, 2000.
5. Sackett DL and others: *Evidence-based medicine: how to practice and teach EBM,* ed 2, New York, 2000, Churchill Livingstone.
6. Towheed TE, Hochberg MC: A systematic review of randomized controlled trials of pharmacological therapy in osteoarthritis of the knee, with an emphasis on trial methodology, *Semin Arthritis Rheum* 26(5):755-770, 1997.
7. U.S. Preventive Services Task Force: *Guide to clinical preventive services,* ed 2, Baltimore, 1996, Williams & Wilkins.
8. Williams JW and others: A systematic review of newer pharmacotherapies for depression in adults: evidence report summary, *Ann Intern Med* 132:743-756, 2000.

# CHAPTER 8

# *Guidelines and Pathways*

## INTRODUCTION

Health-care entities ranging from hospitals to managed-care organizations seem to rely more and more on clinical guidelines and care pathways. Such documents are designed to address not merely a single evidence-based decision but rather a whole segment of the management of a particular type of patient, such as those with community-acquired pneumonia, diabetes, or depression. The motivation for this reliance includes issues such as cost savings, outcomes improvement, and medical error reduction. Creating a care-management pathway is a daunting task.

The use of the terms *guideline, pathway,* and *algorithm* have become confused and inconsistent in recent years, so this discussion begins with clear definitions of each.

### Algorithms

Algorithms form the most elemental aspect of practice-management literature. Typically an algorithm represents a set of detailed instructions used to carry out a specific task. The task may be diagnostic or therapeutic. Examples of algorithms include instructions to implement anticoagulation with heparin (initial dose, maintenance dose, frequency of blood test monitoring, adjustments to previous dose, and so forth) or insertion of central venous catheters (skin preparation technique, trimming of the catheter, preferred dressing). Although an algorithm may contain several decision points, it is basically a step-by-step instruction sheet for a complex but specific task. In many ways, an algorithm is similar to a checklist, although branch points may be included in the algorithm. If patient care were a gourmet meal, an algorithm would be the recipe for dessert.

### Clinical Guidelines

A clinical guideline is a standardized set of recommendations for the management of patients with a specific clinical condition, including presumptions about certain decisions, the relative importance of various outcomes, and the validity of the reviewed clinical evidence on which the recommendations are based.

A clinical guideline usually is created because the care of a specific condition within the medical community of interest has been shown to exhibit one of the following patterns:

1. Wide variation from physician to physician
2. Substandard outcomes
3. Excessive cost

Based on a thorough review of the best available evidence (subject to thoughtful critical appraisal), participants in the clinical community agree on a standard of care that is widely acceptable. The process of development is designed to build consensus among the key stakeholders in the guideline to enhance compliance. When the best evidence is inadequate to address a specific point in the guideline, the recommendation often is either to leave that step to the discretion of the physician or to adhere to standard practice.

To extend the gourmet-meal analogy introduced in the algorithm discussion, a clinical guideline would explain how to serve the entire meal. The guideline would instruct the host to serve the appetizer; if the gourmand prefers chicken, serve white wine; otherwise serve red wine; serve the salad; serve the entrée; if the plate is emptied quickly, offer seconds; if not, wait until everyone has finished; then serve dessert; and so on.

**Reflection of Opinions within Guidelines** By specifying the decision points, defining the possible choices, and specifying precisely what to do once a decision is made, a guideline virtually always includes (implicitly or explicitly) a degree of opinion reflecting the bias of the authors, however well-meaning it may be. To refer to the gourmet-meal example again, not everyone likes white wine with chicken.

| Example |
| --- |

A clinical guideline about the treatment of abnormal tuberculosis skin tests contains a decision point that depends on a patient's age. If the patient is age 35 or older, no treatment is given for a positive tuberculin skin test, whereas for those patients younger than age 35, antibiotic treatment is recommended.

The data on which this recommendation is based reflects an increasing incidence of liver toxicity resulting from the antibiotic in older patients, compared with younger patients, and such evidence is of questionable validity.[5] No randomized controlled trials (RCTs) or cohort outcome trials exist to compare positive reactors age 36 who elect to take the antibiotic to those age 35 who do not take the preventive treatment; no consideration is given to the patient's opinion about a very small risk of serious liver problems, compared with a small but larger risk of the development of future active tuberculosis. Although the guideline is sensible by the value system of its authors, it may or may not be sensible for use on an individual patient.

An interesting confirmation of the embedded opinions inherent in guidelines is found in a recent study of the management of atrial fibrillation with anticoagulation, a seemingly iron-clad plan given recent data.[6] The standard guideline was compared with a decision-analysis approach through use of the same evidence, the only exception being that in the decision analysis, each patient was directed to provide subjective preferences for the various possible outcomes. Although decision analysis is discussed in detail in a later chapter, suffice it to say that the article demonstrated that almost half of all patients treated according to the guideline would have been served better (according to their own value systems) with a different course of action.

This most recent example was not a question of patients making scientific or clinical decisions, only of patients expressing their feelings about the various consequences of their decisions (for example, stroke, death, anticoagulant therapy). The example does not prove the guideline "wrong" in terms of mortality and morbidity, but it shows that the authors' perceptions and judgments about morbidity can differ from those of many patients.

Clinical guidelines contain elements of systematic reviews; indeed the clinical guideline is based ideally on the results of a systematic review of the evidence. Unlike a systematic review, however, a guideline does more than present and appraise the best available evidence; it proceeds to incorporate that evidence into a series of steps and recommendations for patient care. This step indeed sets up a profound difference between the clinical guideline and the systematic review and often is the source of much controversy among clinicians. A key point to ensure compliance with a guideline is to gain the consensus of its potential users; this step generally is performed not because of disagreement about the underlying evidence but rather because of a desire about how to implement it.

The American College of Physicians (ACP) in its *Annals of Internal Medicine* has adopted the commendable practice of presenting a separate systematic review to accompany each of its guidelines. Aside from raising the reader's confidence in the fundamental evidence on which the guideline is based, this process allows each reader to separate fact from strategy and opinion.

**Political and Practical Implications of Guidelines**  Once I was asked to comply with a well-meaning but ill-conceived guideline for the treatment of pneumonia. The task force that created the guideline worked diligently to review the available literature (but did not critically appraise it very well), and also studied the local experience with this condition for possible additional opportunities to improve care. Unfortunately, their analysis turned up several associations that stretched the limits of plausibility. For example, the guideline included the following recommendations:

1. All patients with an arterial oxygen saturation concentrations less than 89% should receive a social-service consultation within 24 hours of admission. (These patients seemed to have longer lengths of stay in the hospital, so the authors believed that this mandate would expedite their discharge and get social service involved early.)

The medical community reacted with common sense rather than blind compliance, noting that naturally sicker patients should have longer hospital stays; that many of these patients were inappropriate candidates for immediate social-service consultations, notwithstanding their poor blood gas results; and that no evidence existed that social-service consultation on the first day of a hospital stay helped reduce the length of stay for any group.

2. All patients who fail to improve within 48 hours of admission should receive a pulmonary-medicine consultation.

This recommendation created skepticism as well. No evidence existed that it improved outcomes, and it offended many physicians, who felt that their judgment as to when to request a consultation was being questioned without valid cause. In addition, the guideline's authors included a number of pulmonologists at the hospital whose practices were not yet full. Many patients' failures to improve within that time frame could have been due to numerous other factors not requiring consultation.

Such unsuccessful attempts at guideline implementation have been repeated many times in the early days of guidelines and continue to occur too often. Creating and implementing a guideline is a major undertaking that requires experience, expertise, and profound understanding of the local medical and political communities.

Therefore each guideline should have a "champion," someone who is respected for knowledge and experience in the field, accepted politically, and has high integrity in the community. As a consensus builder, the champion often can anticipate and prevent many of the problems described in the previous discussion.

**Guideline Validation** An important aspect of guideline implementation is the collection of baseline outcome data to provide information about how patients are faring under the existing, preguideline standard of care. Periodically the effects of the new guidelines should be measured carefully and compared against the previous benchmark data. If the quality of care improves and the costs are acceptable or if the quality is essentially unchanged and the costs decrease, the guideline can be used with confidence and promoted widely. On the other hand, if the quality diminishes, the guideline should be reassessed.

The concept of testing a guideline after implementation should be part of the initial guideline creation process. Few arguments for compliance with a guideline are more convincing than a sound trial showing improved outcomes, with stable or reduced costs in the community of interest.

## Pathways

Algorithms and guidelines both are relatively focused in their scope. At the most global level of care-management literature is the clinical pathway, sometimes referred to as a *critical pathway.** Pathways combine several practice guidelines (each of which may contain algorithms) into a set of recommendations that generally cover a longer period of time than does a clinical practice guideline. Depending on the clinical context, a pathway may, for example, track a patient through an initial diagnosis, subsequent management, rehabilitation, and follow-up planning. This type of document is common in managed-care settings and other enterprises in which such global standardization is considered beneficial.

Returning one last time to the gourmet-meal analogy, if an algorithm is the recipe for dessert and a guideline is a branching set of suggestions used to serve the entire meal, a pathway would be the proposed plan for the entire evening's festivities. The pathway would instruct the host to greet the guests; ask the butler to handle storing the coats and hats; serve cocktails at 8:00 PM and then proceed to the meal (referring to the appropriate guidelines for the preparation and serving of the meal and the appropriate algorithms for the cooking of the dessert). After dinner, the pathway would instruct the user to serve brandy and cigars (consulting the mixology guideline) and expedite charming conversation (consulting the algorithm for discussion of, for example, the Green Bay Packers). Note that guidelines and algorithms are ingredients *inside* the pathway.

Like guidelines, pathways should be tested against "usual" care before they are accepted for general use.

Figure 8.1 depicts the relationship of the previously discussed issues in the management of diabetes (grossly simplified to illustrate the point). Because pathways are largely institution- or community-specific and algorithms are entirely task driven, the following discussion focuses on clinical guidelines. Evidence within guidelines is drawn on most heavily to justify recommended courses of action. Readers desiring further detail about the process used to develop and implement pathways and guidelines are referred to the articles by Ellrodt and colleagues.[1-2]

---

*The reasons for the use of the term *critical* are unclear. Most pathways do not involve critical care, and the clinical scenarios they address are no more or less critical to patient care in general than many others. Perhaps the term inadvertently describes the reception such pathways often receive among their intended users.

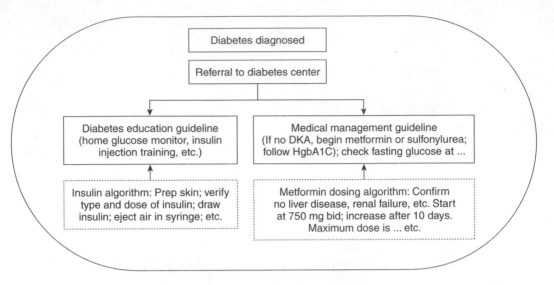

**Figure 8.1**   A simplified critical pathway for the treatment of diabetes. The pathway *(oval)* can be composed of guidelines *(solid rectangles)* linked by recommended paths of action; algorithms *(dotted rectangles)* provide specific instructions for implementation of parts of a guideline.

## Protocols

The word *protocol* is used in numerous ways in case-management literature; it seems to lack a rigid definition in this context. Often the term refers to what might be considered an algorithm (for example, a protocol for heparin administration), but in a number of cases it seems to refer to a guideline (for example, a protocol for diabetic ketoacidosis management). *Protocol* is mentioned in this discussion for the sake of completeness; readers are advised to be alert to its use and classify it as one or another of the three categories described previously (that is, an algorithm, a clinical guideline, or a pathway).

## Advantages of Clinical Guidelines

Proponents of the widespread use of clinical guidelines note several possible advantages to their use, as follows:

- Reduction in medical errors of *omission,* such as a failure to order a specific treatment or test
- Reduction in medical errors of *commission,* such as drug dosage errors
- Increase in efficiency due to widespread familiarity with the standard of care among clinicians and support staff
- Potential cost savings if a guideline promotes decreased use of interventions with no proven value for the patient
- Decrease in length of hospital stay or in duration of illness

## Disadvantages of Clinical Guidelines

Among the disadvantages to the use of clinical guidelines are the following:

- Potential for harm to patients when inappropriately rigid guidelines fail to account for individual variation
- Loss of physician autonomy and innovation in the care of patients
- Dissonance if the conscientious provider fails to agree with the contents of a guideline
- Cumbersome and confusing logistical problems when several entities each promote a different guideline for the same clinical condition (hospitals, managed-care groups, national specialty societies, federal agencies)
- Possibly increased legal liability for both the provider and the sponsoring entity when the undesirable outcomes occur despite proper adherence to the guideline (or when undesirable outcomes occur despite appropriate care that does not happen to follow the guideline)
- Forced acceptance of the implied value judgments inherent in a guideline

A guideline (or pathway) is only as strong or as feeble as the evidence on which it is based and the flexibility, clinical experience, and practical wisdom used to apply it. The evidence-based decision maker will do well to appraise carefully every guideline and pathway that the practitioner is requested to adopt. Where flaws are apparent, the practitioner should provide the important feedback required and deviate from the guideline, if necessary, to provide the best care for the patient in question. When an excellent guideline is provided, the practitioner may consider it a great time saver and quality safety net.

# RETRIEVING GUIDELINES

## Master Evidence Question

The Master Evidence Question for guidelines is as follows:

> *Is this guideline based on suitable evidence, sound logic, and appropriate opinions, and is it feasible in my setting?*

The usual search strategies described in previous chapters are designed to find primary evidence from clinical trials. Guidelines are often the result of systematic reviews and consensus panels and thus may be missed. Broad-based, preappraised literature compendia such as Best Evidence occasionally include guidelines and are a good place to start. In many cases, though, the user must to turn to MEDLINE and specialized guideline repositories, as addressed in the following section.

**Searching MEDLINE for Guidelines** Users first should supplement their usual search strategy with a search on the topic, accompanied by the phrase

*AND (guideline OR pathway)*. MEDLINE recognizes the specific publication type "practice guideline," providing another applicable filter.

> **Example**

> **Pass 1:** Pneumonia AND (guideline OR pathway)
> *Comment:* This search retrieved 244 articles in PubMed, including many judged clearly irrelevant from the title alone, perhaps because they used the word *guideline* or *pathway* in a different context within the abstract or text.

> **Pass 2:** #1 AND practice guideline
> *Comment:* This entry reduced the list to 71 citations, a workable number, quite a few of which were relevant.

As with many search strategies, the previous example has not been validated scientifically. It has, however, proven reliable and efficient in my experience.

## Guideline Repositories

A number of databases specialize in the listing of guidelines, many of which are not included in MEDLINE. Among these sources are the following:

- The United States government's Agency for Healthcare Research and Quality (AHRQ) sponsors the National Guideline Clearinghouse at the website www.guideline.gov. This site bills itself as "a public resource for evidence based clinical practice guidelines." It features a searchable database and the ability to maintain each user's personal selection of guidelines for future reference. The resources include the AHRQ's own guidelines on a wide range of topics, as well as guidelines from the American Medical Association and the American Association of Health Plans. A useful feature is the ability to compare two or more guidelines on the same topic through a structured table that lists summaries of the guidelines' components side by side.
- The National Library of Medicine maintains the Health Services/Technology Assessment Text (HSTAT) at http://text.nlm.nih.gov/ftrs/gateway. This repository by its own description from the preceding website includes the following information:

    . . . clinical practice guidelines, quick-reference guides for clinicians, consumer brochures, and evidence reports sponsored by the Agency for Health Care Policy and Research (AHCPR); AHCPR technology assessment reports; National Institutes of Health (NIH) consensus development conference and technology assessment reports; NIH Warren G. Magnuson Clinical Center research protocols; HIV/AIDS Treatment Information Service (ATIS) resource documents; Substance Abuse and Mental Health Services Administration, Center for Substance Abuse Treatment (SAMHSA/CSAT) treatment improvement protocols; and the Public Health Service (PHS) Preventive Services Task Force Guide to Clinical Preventive Services.

- The ACP has a website at www.acponline.org/sci-policy/guidelines. This site contains a compendium of guidelines published in the *Annals of Internal Medicine.* Useful features include full-text listing of the entire contents of the published guideline. Of interest to evidence-based medicine (EBM) advocates is that the *Annals of Internal Medicine* generally presents ACP-sanctioned guidelines in the context of an accompanying systematic review of the topic, many of which are quite rigorous. Thus users can view both the primary evidence and the guideline that is derived from it.

Many other specialty organizations publish guidelines of varying quality. Honing the skills necessary to appraise these guidelines is especially important because many guidelines are based on little more than the consensus of a panel of physicians whose skill in appraising evidence may be considerably inferior to the physician seeking the evidence. The air of authority surrounding "official" guidelines should not deter any practitioner from appraising them very carefully.

## JUDGING THE SUITABILITY OF GUIDELINES

### Preparations

Before appraising the validity and applicability of a guideline or pathway, performance of a preliminary assessment of its *raison d' etre,* or its "reason for being," is important.

First the practitioner should assess the motivation of the group that generated the guideline. Although blatant self-interest is rarely a factor in guidelines from reputable groups, subtle influences possibly may affect objectivity from time to time. Without adopting a cynical approach, the practitioner should remain aware of funding sources, political agendas, and potential commercial profit motives. If such influences are considered early in the appraisal process, the practitioner may be able to anticipate trends and directions in the guidelines that raise concerns. In addition, the practitioner should remain aware of selection bias if the purity of the sponsor's motivation comes under scrutiny; although the presented evidence may be valid, verification of whether contradictory evidence of comparable validity also was considered may be necessary.

Furthermore, the practitioner should remain cautious about single-authored guidelines and pathways. Although they are not inherently unsound, a likely finding is that participation of all the necessary stakeholders has not been achieved. Again, a guideline is not a systematic review; it is the implementation of patient-care recommendations based on an evidence review, which usually requires a group of people.

### Applicability

Because guidelines are highly focused, the applicability of a guideline to the patient in question usually is clear. In fact a basic applicability criterion is an explicit definition of the patient population for which the guideline is intended. If the practitioner cannot determine the basic elements of applicability from a guideline, that source should not be used. The disease type, age, clinical context, and other basic conditions of the population should be crystal clear.

If the guideline might apply to the patient in question, the practitioner then should assess whether it might be beneficial. If that practitioner's usual patient care follows the guideline already, further appraisal is unnecessary. If not, the practitioner should examine whether the discrepancies have the potential to improve outcomes or efficiency. For example, if the only difference between the usual care and that called for by the guideline is a minor switch to an equivalent drug, the practitioner either may follow the guideline's recommendation or continue the current practice.

On the other hand, if adhering to the guideline would render important or systematic changes to the usual patient care, the practitioner should appraise its validity thoroughly. In such cases that physician may well learn valuable information, and the patient may benefit.

## Validity

The following points should be used to assess the validity of a guideline:[4]

1. Is a problem truly present? The authors should clarify why the guideline was created (for example, cost, quality, length of stay, or quality of life). A fine guideline may be of little consequence if the condition it addresses is already being handled effectively and efficiently in the community in question.
2. Are the flow and logic of the guideline clinically sensible and complete; do they "feel" natural?
3. Does the guideline include all the anticipated branch points and likely outcomes usually encountered? Readers may discover a hint to problems in this area if they find themselves making statements such as, "Yes, but what if . . . ," or "That's fine, but what about . . ."
4. Are the recommendations justified by valid and applicable evidence, explicitly cited and appraised?
5. Are personal preferences for relevant decisions taken into account? In other words, phrasing such as, "for patients preferring surgery over radiation, proceed to . . ." or, "for patients for whom this risk is not acceptable, proceed to . . ." may provide clues. In any case the flow for decisions that might depend on a patient's personal values should be analyzed, and the guideline should recognize these factors by allowing for variation to reflect such values.
6. Where the guideline assigns a specific course of action to a given situation, are the authors' judgments consistent with those of the physician and the patient? For example, if the guideline calls for omission of a diagnostic test because a potentially fatal condition is "only" 2% likely, should

the physician accept that judgment? Or, by contrast, if a guideline calls for performance of an expensive or uncomfortable test for a nonfatal disease because it is 2% likely, should the physician agree with that judgment?

Most importantly, given the immediate and sometimes unyielding impact of a guideline on actual practice patterns, perhaps all practitioners should adapt a higher standard yet: Every important guideline should be compared in a randomized, controlled fashion against "usual care," and only after it is deemed safe and effective should it be adopted. Practitioners readily accept such a standard for new drugs, so why should the bar be lowered for guidelines?

This recommendation is not judged extreme, considering that in 1993 the American Thoracic Society issued a clinical guideline for the care of community-acquired pneumonia. Gleason and colleagues[3] tested this guideline in a prospective multicenter cohort study that analyzed subjects who were either treated in accordance with the guidelines or were not. One subset (patients older than 60 years of age) in the guideline-consistent group had a 1000% higher antibiotic cost, with outcomes that were not superior to the guideline-inconsistent group. The study's authors corrected the results for severity of illness and other necessary factors. Although this study was not a direct prospective comparison of guideline-directed versus usual-care cohorts, it did raise questions about the importance of the validation of guidelines after they are generated.

As a practicing physician, I am philosophically accepting of clinical guidelines if they expedite adherence to evidence-based care. In practice, however, many guidelines that have been proposed have lacked one or more of the key suitability criteria described in the previous discussion.[7] Furthermore, even "valid" guidelines generally rely on a collection of individual bits of evidence combined in a particular sequence and decision context that has not been tested as a collective "whole." Knowing that a guideline has been validated by a sound outcome study would increase markedly my confidence in adhering to it, and thus my compliance with it. For this reason, prospective validation should be the gold standard for a clinical guideline.

## Master Decision Question for Guidelines

The Master Decision Question for guidelines is as follows:

> *Will using this guideline improve patient care or improve efficiency without diminishing the quality of patient care?*

The inherent logic of this question bears little discussion. Perhaps the only point worth emphasizing is that a guideline that improves efficiency alone (without affecting or compromising patient care) should receive the practitioner's full attention in this era of limited resources. To reject automatically any guideline that fails to improve clinical outcomes is tempting, but to do so if it can save money, reduce hospital stays, or expedite work flow seems irresponsible unless the burden of adherence is very high.

## GUIDELINE IMPLEMENTATION ISSUES

Example

Imagine that you are faced with a guideline disseminated by a respected group of your peers regarding the treatment of asthma in your hospital. The guideline is accompanied by a thorough and up-to-date list of primary evidence, each piece of which has been appraised in a logical and conscientious manner. In your hospital, both the need for mechanical ventilation and the length of hospital stays have exceeded the national benchmarks, and this observation motivated the creation of the guideline. The task force that created the guideline is composed of five physicians, two nurses, and one patient with asthma.

Unfortunately, the implementation of this guideline involved no more than a somewhat abrupt announcement that the process would commence the following month. Although you feel a bit excluded by this process, you recognize that the potential benefit to your patients is important and you are willing to give it a try.

Shortly after the implementation of the guideline, you are having lunch in the physicians' lounge. A colleague joins you, clearly distraught by an incident that occurred that morning. She says she admitted a patient with asthma and wrote her usual orders. A few minutes later, she received a phone call from the head nurse, who stated the following information:

*"We don't administer that medicine any longer; it is not in the guideline."*

The medicine in question was an inhaler essentially equivalent to that called for by the guideline. Furthermore, the patient had received a chest radiograph ("per the guideline") shortly after admission, a test the physician had not ordered because one had been performed in the office less than 1 hour before the patient's admission.

This example illustrates the difficulties involved in the implementation of even a valid, applicable guideline. The best defense against such errors includes the following measures:

1. Widely include representatives from all possible stakeholders early in the process. Create a robust guideline using all the tools of EBM.
2. Educate the providers tactfully, as individually as possible, using medical evidence freely. Physicians want to do the right thing primarily for medical, not economic, reasons.
3. When possible, ensure that adherence does not create financial disincentives; this challenge is difficult outside managed-care settings, but creative administrators can help.

4. If a pathway or guideline calls for the rendering of traditional physician services by nonphysicians, take measures to communicate with the physicians frequently so that continuity of care is disrupted as little as possible.
5. Use pilot implementations in small, highly structured settings first, refine the process based on those experiences, and expand it incrementally, learning as the process progresses.
6. For remedies to problems generated by the new guideline, look to the victims—those who were affected adversely by the flaw. Correct the problems and be persistent; do not abandon efforts simply because problems arise early.
7. Measure the outcomes before, during, and after implementation. The best way to improve compliance is to show that the guideline worked so that doubters become believers over time.

A widespread belief exists that physicians fail to comply with guidelines because of political or economic motivations. The evidence suggests that this belief is not the case. A retrospective study examined the implementation of a guideline for management of chest pain in low-risk individuals.[2] The guideline was validated carefully before implementation, and a 2-day hospital stay was shown to be safe and effective. The authors' analysis concluded that in only 16% of subjects was the guideline disregarded because of the physician's explicit refusal to accept it. In the other cases, factors such as hospital inefficiency, changes in patient status during admission, or errors in classification of patients were the culprits. This example demonstrates that most physicians will adhere to a sound guideline if they are given the ability to do so.

## SUMMARY

If a robust systematic review is the best of all worlds where evidence is concerned, then a sound clinical guideline has the same potential when it is applied to the overall management of a specific disorder. Most physicians accept a useful and validated clinical guideline as a tool to ensure that their care is efficient, thorough, and effective. Just as aircraft pilots rely throughout their careers on checklists, physicians can use guidelines as a first line of defense against errors of omission and commission.

To extend this flight analogy, the most complete checklist in the aviation industry cannot teach a pilot how to fly an airplane. Such is the case in medicine. A practicing physician might embrace high-quality, validated guidelines as a wonderful means to distill large amounts of evidence and community values about the care of a disease; however, the actual rendering of care necessitates an enormous amount of additional judgment, sensitivity, common sense, experience, and, decision-making skills. A great guideline is a powerful tool—but only in the hands of a great physician.

# REFERENCES

1. Ellrodt AG and others: Evidence-based disease management, *JAMA* 278:1687-1692, 1997.
2. Ellrodt AG and others: Measuring and improving physician compliance with clinical practice guidelines: a controlled interventional trial, *Ann Intern Med* 122(4):277-282, 1995.
3. Gleason PP and others: Medical outcomes and antimicrobial costs with the use of the American Thoracic Society guidelines for outpatients with community-acquired pneumonia, *JAMA* 278:32-39, 1997.
4. Hayward RSA and others: Users' guides to the medical literature. VIII. How to use clinical practice guidelines. A. Are the recommendations valid? *JAMA* 274:570-574, 1995.
5. Nolan CM: Community-wide implementation of targeted testing for and treatment of latent tuberculosis infection, *Clin Infect Dis* 29(4):880-887, 1999.
6. Protheroe J and others: The impact of patients' preferences on the treatment of atrial fibrillation: observational study of patient based decision analysis, *BMJ* 320(7246):1380-1384, 2000.
7. Wilson MC and others: Users' guides to the medical literature. VIII. How to use clinical practice guidelines. B. What are the recommendations and will they help you in caring for your patients? *JAMA* 274:1630-1632, 1995.

# CHAPTER 9

# *Decision Analysis*

## INTRODUCTION

Previous chapters have focused on the many basic elements of decision analysis. For example, Chapters 3 and 4, respectively, demonstrated how to estimate an action threshold (AT) for a treatment-diagnosis diad and how to predict disease likelihood from diagnostic tests. Using these two concepts, readers were able to perform fundamental decision analyses.

> **Example**

> For a patient with a large aneurysm of the abdominal aorta, you use your evidence-retrieval skills to learn the annual risk that it will rupture, which would cause catastrophic outcomes. You also learn that surgery reduces this risk substantially but that surgery itself carries a risk of stroke, heart attack, death, and other complications. By comparing the frequency and impacts of these outcomes, you derive an AT as follows:

$$AT = \frac{\text{frequency} \times \text{impact [of surgical complications]}}{\text{frequency} \times \text{impact [of reduction in risk of rupture]}}$$

> In so doing, you have performed a decision analysis, incorporating the evidence and the patient's values (in the impact component). Your AT score reflects the level of confidence you must have in the diagnosis before you will advise the patient to undergo surgery. If the AT is 0.1, even a 10% likelihood of this diagnosis would warrant surgery.

Decision skills such as those presented in this example are profoundly important in daily practice. Still, some scenarios are far too complex to allow such off-the-cuff analysis. For example, three or more initial options may exist, each of which leads to several possibilities depending on the individual outcomes. Quick mental tracking of all the possibilities becomes impossible.

Methodologic tools exist to solve such complex decision analyses, and important papers are published every year that use such formal analysis. This chapter introduces the core concepts behind the steps of an analysis so that readers can both appraise their suitability and appreciate their power and limitations.

# *Components of a Decision Analysis*

## UNDERSTANDING FORMAL DECISION ANALYSIS

This section details the mechanics of the decision tree, a tool used in most formal decision analyses found in the literature. Although other tools exist, decision trees best exemplify the concepts of medical decision analysis. Readers who would rather not delve into the details but simply glean the "bottom line" of the decision tree are advised to consult the section entitled, "Interpreting a Decision Analysis" in Section Three. However, appraisal of decision analyses is difficult without a basic understanding of the process. For readers interested in further information about this decision-making tool, Detsky and colleagues[1] have written a detailed tutorial on the performance of a decision analysis.

*Example*

Suppose you are trying to select an architect to build your dream house. You have narrowed the list to two finalists, whose backgrounds reveal the following:

Architect 1 is very temperamental. When in a good mood (which occurs about half the time), she produces fabulous work. Her better houses are among the best you have ever seen, and she refuses to design the same house twice. When she is in a bad mood, her houses are mediocre.

Architect 2 is as solid as a rock. She rarely produces extraordinary houses (5% of the time), but the remainder of her houses are decent (that is, better than mediocre).

You are putting up a lot of money for this project, so you decide to analyze your choice more carefully. Figure 9.1 details one way you might depict the situation.

Figure 9.1 illustrates the decision as a tree diagram. The initial choice is at the left, shown as a small square with two choices branching from it. This type of node is called a *decision node* because the path to be taken is under the user's control (that is, a conscious decision).

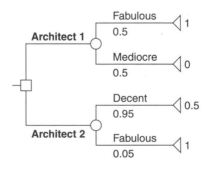

**Figure 9.1**   The architect decision in a diagram. The scenario unfolds left to right; the outcome is listed above each branch, with its likelihood listed beneath the branch. Note the decision node *(open square)*, the chance nodes *(open circles)*, and the terminal nodes *(open triangles)*.

Moving from either of the two decision branches to the next "generation" of branching, the diagram shows the likelihood of each type of house, based on evidence about the history of each architect as noted in the previous example. These nodes are depicted as circles and are called *chance nodes* because their relative likelihoods are presumed to be based on fixed evidence. No decision is made at the chance nodes, but the evidence can be used to predict the relative likelihood of each outcome.

Finally, each branch reaches its natural conclusion based on the preceding path; these are called *terminal nodes* and are shown as triangles.

The decision now is diagrammed neatly. From beginning to end the scenario can unfold in any of four paths, depending on the initial choice and the likelihood of the possible outcomes. All that is missing is some sort of judgment score about how good or bad each of the terminal nodes might be. These values (empirically assigned based on the user's opinions) are known as *utilities* and are shown to the right of the triangular terminal nodes in Figure 9.1.

## Utilities

Previous chapters have discussed the concept of impacts, describing them as numbers from 0 to 1 that reflect how important an outcome is to a patient. Whether the outcome is good or bad does not matter, only how important the outcome is. Formal decision analysis (including decision trees) uses an analogous concept known as *utilities*. Like impacts, utilities reflect subjective value judgments on the part of the decision maker. Also like impacts, utilities use a 0-to-1 scale. *Unlike* impacts, however, utilities are directional in that the higher the number, the better the outcome; conversely, the lower the number, the worse the outcome.

Another ground rule applies to the use of utilities. Within the scenario under analysis, the best of all outcomes (regardless of what the "best" might be) is assigned a score of 1, and the worst is assigned a 0. Every other outcome receives an intermediate score reflecting its relative and proportional goodness or badness in comparison with the two extremes.

Estimating utilities is complex and controversial. Numerous techniques used to assist patients in the task have been devised, including "standard gambles" and other games that strive to promote consistency. Readers are referred to the references[1,2,4] for further detail. Suffice it to say that in many ways the bottom line is that the number should reflect what the decision maker actually feels, and the analyst's role is to provide the decision maker with complete information and neutral coaching to ensure that the values are rational and consistent.

## Solving the Decision Tree

Once the values for each branch and terminal node are completed, the tree may be "solved." Solving a tree in decision-analysis jargon is known as "folding"

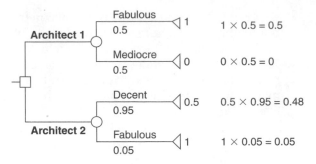

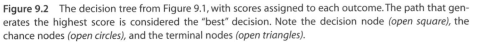

**Figure 9.2** The decision tree from Figure 9.1, with scores assigned to each outcome. The path that generates the highest score is considered the "best" decision. Note the decision node *(open square)*, the chance nodes *(open circles)*, and the terminal nodes *(open triangles)*.

or "rolling back." It is simple, if a bit tedious with larger trees, and is done as follows:

1. For each terminal node, its utility is multiplied by the probability of the branch immediately preceding it.
2. The value obtained in step 1 becomes a new "utility" for the node preceding (to the left of) the branch in question. This new utility then is multiplied by the probability for the branch preceding *it*, and so forth, until the origin of the tree is reached.
3. The final mathematic product becomes the score for that "path" from start to terminal node. In jargon this score is the *expected utility* for that path.

The path with the highest expected utility becomes the "best" decision. Figure 9.2 shows the tree with the expected utilities calculated for each path. In this case the first path (architect 1; fabulous) has the highest score, with 0.5. The third path (architect 2; decent) is a close second at 0.48; even a slight change in the utility for this path might have turned the tables. Given that the judgment is a subjective at best, the analyst of this decision tree should have some uneasiness about such a close call.

Several computer programs exist to help users diagram and solve decision trees. A program called *DATA* (Treeage, Williamstown, Mass.) is a good example. Solving decision trees becomes too cumbersome to perform mentally after only a few sets of branches, and even more calculations are required if the assumptions change—the "what if" analyses. Programs such as DATA allow the analyst to perform complicated analyses and test them under a variety of assumptions. However, even the most complex of these programs relies on the basic principles described in the previous discussion.

Figure 9.3 illustrates a computer-generated tree for the treatment of prostatism. The utilities at the right are assigned to variables rather than being entered as absolute numbers; the lower-left listing shows the currently assigned values. The roll-back for this tree takes a second or two and can be repeated under a wide range of value assumptions. Sensitivity analyses (discussed in

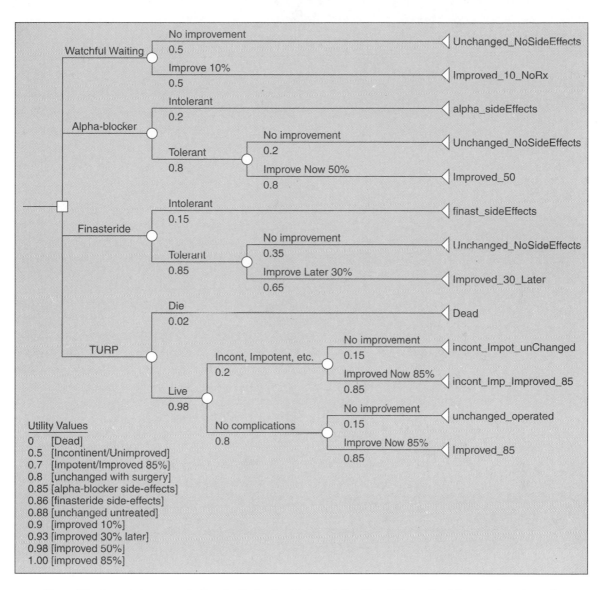

**Figure 9.3** A computer-generated tree for the treatment of prostatism. The utilities on the right are assigned to variables, not entered as absolute numbers. The lower-left listing illustrates the currently assigned values.

Section Three) also are performed automatically, allowing for stringent testing of the tree's conclusions.

This chapter's treatment of decision analysis to this point has been highly mechanical. Section Three of this chapter discusses how to apply these mechanics to patient decisions. First, however, Section Two focuses on how to retrieve and appraise decision analyses in much the same way traditional types of evidence are retrieved and appraised.

# *Decision Analysis as Evidence*

## DECISION ANALYSIS AS EVIDENCE

### Master Evidence Question

The Master Evidence Question for decision analysis is as follows:

> *Does this decision analysis identify an optimal management sequence based on sound evidence, reasonable logic, and sensible utilities?*

Now that the anatomy and physiology of a decision tree have been addressed, the practitioner can answer this question by ensuring that its components are well structured and the values used by the study's authors are acceptable for the patient at hand.

### Controversy about Decision Analysis

A decision analysis (or tree) is only a mathematic model. In the business world, where the technique originated, utilities are replaced with dollars. The cost and profit of an outcome are analogous to the beneficial and adverse outcomes of interest. In such a context the "best path" is simply that which yields the highest profit based on the probabilities provided. Under such conditions the technique can be proved useful; its quantitative validity is not in question.

In clinical medicine the decision tree is quite another story. The cost of an adverse outcome is measured in human suffering, and a beneficial outcome is measured essentially in terms of prevented suffering. Critics of decision analysis in medicine have questioned whether the entire premise fails because of this subjectivity. A few targeted questions can help practitioners inspect this and other criticisms further.

#### Does the Subjective Nature of Utilities Render Them Unsuitable for Mathematic Analysis?

Clearly, the decision tree is not a precise, engineering-quality parameter. However, with proper use of survey data and techniques such as the standard gamble and time trade-off,* acceptable consistency can be obtained for utilities in a formal analysis. In individual scenarios, patients usually express confidence in the relative utilities they assign to outcomes within a particular situation.

#### Can Definitive Decisions Be Made from a Decision Analysis When the Underlying Numbers Are So Imprecise?

*Definitive* is the key word in this question; if it is intended to mean "sure to result in the best outcome," then the answer is *no:* Decision analysis cannot provide that answer. On the other hand, if *definitive* implies the "best bet" of all

---

*Standard gamble is a technique in which a patient is asked to choose between a certain outcome on the one hand and a varying likelihood of two other outcomes on the other. By adjusting the probabilities appropriately the interviewer can "force" a situation in which the choice is a toss-up. This state reveals the patient's "true" utility on a numeric scale. Time trade-off involves questioning of a patient as to how long that individual would accept in a state of good health, compared with a fixed length of time spent in poor health. In appropriate clinical scenarios this technique also allows for the quantification of how a patient feels about a health outcome (see Sox and colleagues[4] for further information).

the outcomes, then the technique indeed can provide guidance. As with all medical decisions, some patients who follow the best path might end up much worse for their efforts, just as some of those who choose the risky path fare very well. This concept is akin to betting on a royal flush in a poker game. The bettor may lose once in a while, but not making the bet at all would be foolish in the long run.

### Is the Difference in Scores between Paths So Slight that Neither Choice Seems Clearly the Best?

Just as small differences in the efficacy of competing treatments are often of no statistical significance, so is the case in decision analysis. If the difference in the expected utility between paths is so small that subtle changes in the underlying assumptions would change their ranking, the final decision is too close to call. A saving grace in many such cases is the technique known as *sensitivity analysis,* which is discussed in more detail in Section Three. It often reveals that as long as Assumption 1 remains below a certain value, then Path A is the best course; however, if the value is higher than that certain value, then Path B is recommended. Still, in some cases the roll-back simply fails to differentiate clearly between (or among) two or more decision paths.

A final reply to general critics of the use of medical decision analysis involves questioning of those critics as to which approach(es) they would advise instead. Typical responses include *experience, intuition, good judgment,* and *common sense.* Although the importance of these qualities should not be underestimated, they seem to be applied best to the creation of a sound decision analysis and the interpretation of its conclusions, rather than as a total alternative solution. No mind can digest and accurately interpret more than just a few variables and competing strategies at once. A decision tree can fill in these gaps.

### Additional Benefits of Decision Analysis

A well-executed decision analysis provides a remarkable means to render explicit all the details and considerations that comprise a complex clinical decision. Depicting them in full detail can reveal insights that are not apparent from a superficial or intuitive consideration.

Decision analysis is highly effective at separating the facts from the values. It "forces" the parties to focus their arguments on either the facts, which can be supported by evidence, or the opinions, about which most analysts can agree to disagree because ultimately the patients' opinions count in any case. Because a given analysis can lead to different conclusions if the utilities vary, practitioners can agree readily on the decision tree while disagreeing on the utilities; many a clinical "argument" is nothing more than such a case. By making this concept clear, a decision tree can render consensus and agreement while still allowing for different conclusions.

I have experienced cases in which the generation of a decision tree has caused parties to reverse their initial positions completely in a very nonthreatening environment. The fact that the "best-path" solution usually remains unknown until the very end of the analysis allows the parties to share their knowledge and experience in creating the tree free of partisan considerations. Only when the tree is acceptable by consensus is the roll-back performed. The effect on those parties who would have selected a different path is usually profound and nonjudgmental.

## RETRIEVING DECISION ANALYSES

Evidence pertaining to decision analyses often turns up in the primary search (for example, for treatment or diagnosis evidence). When preappraised evidence sources are used, the keyword search usually finds any decision analyses right away.

In MEDLINE the process is a bit more complex. Filters that restrict the search to randomized controlled trials (RCTs) may either miss decision analyses or lose them in the shuffle. Because decision analyses are not RCTs or cohort studies, such filters are not effective. For example, a standard therapy search for *pulmonary embolus AND (random\* or therap\*)* retrieved more than 5500 citations; pass 2 yielded more than 400. Neither pass "caught" an important decision article—a prospective cohort study based on a decision model, albeit not a formal decision analysis.[5]

To remedy this flaw in the standard search models, those evidence scenarios that are good candidates for decision analysis should be identified and the search strategy modified appropriately. For example, scenarios in which many competing treatment and diagnostic options exist or in which the natural sequence of management involves more than two steps are good prospects for a decision analysis.

The following strategy is recommended when decision analyses are being sought specifically. Note that no MEDLINE publication type exists that corresponds closely to decision analysis, and no qualitative assessment of this strategy has been performed. The user should begin by performing the usual search for primary diagnostic or therapeutic evidence and then perform the following additional search to locate any decision analyses missed in the first search:

**Pass 1:** Keywords AND decision AND analy\*
**Pass 2:** #1 AND utility

Pass 1 should locate the decision analyses pertaining to that topic, whereas pass 2 should filter such "self-described" decision analysis that are in fact less quantitative sources.

### Example

**Pass 1:** atrial fibrillation AND anticoagulation AND decision AND analy\*
*Results:* 15 citations
*Comment:* The low citation yield enables a full scan of the retrieved articles, at least a handful of which appear to be true decision analyses

(that is, from their titles). The remainder are clearly not, although the search terms obviously are used somewhere in their text.

**Pass 2:** #1 AND utility

*Results:* One article remains, a true decision analysis.

*Comment:* The article in question is a fascinating study in which standard treatment guidelines for atrial fibrillation in the elderly are compared with the results of a formal, individualized decision analysis through use of patient-by-patient utility assessment (which uses the time trade-off method) and accepted evidence for the risk of various outcomes. The article shows that the guidelines went *against the patient's best interest* (as defined by the decision model) in almost half the patients studied![3] (This article was alluded to in the chapter on guidelines [Chapter 8]; now that decision analysis has been discussed, the powerful effects of patient preferences become clear.)

## JUDGING THE SUITABILITY OF A DECISION ANALYSIS

Because decision analysis is a complex tool with technical details that may reach beyond the expertise of many readers (akin to meta-analysis in this regard), a certain degree of faith must be placed in the editorial staff of the publishing journal, as well as commentators of the article. Nonetheless, many elements of the decision analysis can be appraised clearly by the motivated practitioner.

### Applicability

#### Are the Patients Like Mine?

From the applicability standpoint, the criteria that might be used for a systematic review apply. Are the patient demographics, stage of disease, and other relevant clinical factors appropriate to the patient in question?

#### Are the Utilities Sensible for My Patient, or Does the Sensitivity Analysis Include Values that My Patient Would Use?

With the knowledge contained in this chapter the practitioner can determine all the outcomes (the terminal nodes) and the utilities associated with them. Next, the practitioner can evaluate whether these numbers are reasonable to begin with and whether they are reasonable for the patient in particular. For any questionable outcomes or utilities the practitioner may ask whether a sensitivity analysis was performed that incorporates those values that the physician and patient judge most appropriate.

Unique to decision analysis is an additional applicability criterion used to examine the utilities the authors have chosen for their final outcomes. These numbers should be consistent with values the physician feels the individual patient might have chosen. Although such judgments are not made easily, identification with the patient of utilities that warrant verification is well worth careful scrutiny before the decision analysis is deemed applicable.

If the previously stated criteria are met, then applicability is likely.

## Validity

### Does the Evidence Used in the Analysis Meet the Customary Validity Criteria for Its Category?

A decision analysis, like a systematic review or a guideline, should identify explicitly the methodology used to retrieve the evidence on which it relies. This methodology includes search strategies, critical appraisal, and criteria used to establish validity. In essence, the practitioner should question whether the evidence meets the same criteria that physician would apply toward the various types of evidence discussed in previous chapters of this book.

### Is the Decision Logic Rational and Complete?

Regarding the logic of the decision tree, the practitioner should "walk through it" from left to right to determine whether all logical options and outcomes are included. If major omissions are found, the entire logic may be invalid. For example, if a decision node calls for selection between observation and surgery but the practitioner knows that medication and radiation are also important considerations, the analysis should be rejected.

### Are Evidence and Utility "Soft Spots" Dealt with through Appropriate Sensitivity Analysis?

The authors of a decision analysis often identify crucial components of the analysis for which definitive evidence is simply not available. In this case the use of a careful sensitivity analysis can provide considerable reassurance as to the validity of the assumptions used; alternatively, it can highlight a weak point in the validity of the analysis. In addition, the probabilities used in the study may be quite valid but may not be applicable to the individual patient; if the sensitivity analysis encompasses a figure that is more suitable for the patient in question, the practitioner's confidence level increases.

Ensuring that a decision analysis holds up under the range of values the practitioner finds acceptable for all the important variables it incorporates is important. This task may not be trivial and often is difficult to glean from complicated tables.

### Has the Analysis Been Validated in a Prospective Study?

This question is largely wishful thinking. Unlike a clinical guideline, decision analyses often are done for the very reason that a prospective study of the topic is unethical, impractical, or otherwise not readily available. Still, if a decision-analysis conclusion is validated by even a small prospective study comparing the strategies it examined, general extrapolation of its conclusions becomes easier.

Figure 9.4 summarizes the appraisal process for decision analyses.

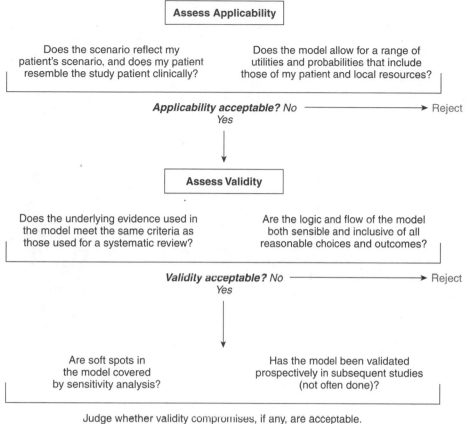

**Figure 9.4** Summary of appraisal criteria for decision analyses. Note that *accept* and *reject* are two extremes of inference as to how closely a study approximates the "truth." Most practitioners' interpretations generally fall somewhere between the two extremes.

# *Helping the Patient Decide*

## USING DECISION ANALYSIS IN MEDICAL DECISION MAKING

### The Master Decision Question

The Master Decision Question for decision analysis is as follows:

*Will use of this analysis identify the best course of action for my patient when two or more competing plans exist?*

The nature of a decision analysis is that it is often applied expressly when more traditional outcomes research is difficult due to impracticality or cost. Nonetheless, under such circumstances a sound decision analysis may provide the best evidence available. If the analysis is subjected to prospective validation, its power increases enormously.

### Sensitivity Analysis

This chapter has shown that numbers fed into a well-designed decision tree can be highly individualized to a given patient. Depending on these numbers, the "best-decision" path may vary. To test how well a decision analysis holds up when its underlying numbers (probabilities and utilities) are varied to accommodate a wide range of clinical scenarios, a technique known as *sensitivity analysis* is used.

This process examines a parameter, the value of which is in question, and verifies it over a selected *range* of values with which the analyst is comfortable. For example, the likelihood of death from carotid endarterectomy is established initially at 1%. A physician may protest that this figure is far too high; a value of 0.5% better reflects local experience. A critic might protest, claiming that the value may be as high as 2% if the low-risk patients are eliminated, and the debate might continue. Thus a range of 0.5% to 2% is ultimately agreed on as encompassing everyone's objections.

If the same best path emerges throughout the entire spectrum of acceptable values, then no one can dispute the robustness of the conclusion. On the other hand, if the best path switches somewhere within that range, the participants must reappraise the data more rigorously rather than arguing about the best path; again the discussion is focused where it should be—on the evidence and not on subjective opinions.

Performing sensitivity analysis also is possible for two or more variables simultaneously. This so-called two-way (or three-way) analysis yields conclusions such as: "The conclusion is valid for values of parameter A below X if parameter B is above Y." Such analyses can be confusing, but they also can prove valuable in selected situations.

Sensitivity analysis provides a powerful tool used to answer objections about the limitations of a decision analysis. It also provides a criterion for critical appraisal of a published decision analysis, as noted in the following discussion.

## INTERPRETING A DECISION ANALYSIS

A formal decision analysis of the type discussed in this chapter consolidates the following components:

- The likelihood of various outcomes based on the best available evidence
- The logical sequence of events based on preceding choices and likelihoods
- The goodness or badness of each possible outcome expressed as a numeric value

Using mathematic values for these components can identify a best path. In this sense the word *best* means the path most likely to result in the optimal combination of frequency and goodness-of-outcome for that patient. This statement implies that the rare occurrence of a bad outcome may count for very little, whereas the very frequent occurrence of a better-than-average outcome might prevail over fairly unlikely occurrences of the best outcome. Considering a best decision (as derived from a decision analysis) as a *weighted* consideration of quality and quantity may be the most accurate description. A couple of examples may clarify this synopsis.

| Examples |

According to reasonable estimations, approximately 1 in 300,000 patients given penicillin will die from the drug. Few clinicians would hesitate to use this drug to treat strep throat. The implied and accepted conclusion is that very rare events, even when severe, should not drive decisions.

A 10% chance of a very bad outcome may be worth accepting in return for a 90% chance of great improvement of a fairly serious ailment. However, as the chances of a very bad outcome increase, a point is reached at which the risk is no longer worth accepting. A decision analysis helps identify that decision point; the best path is the path that best describes the risks and benefits a patient is willing to accept and trade off.

The best path of a decision analysis applies only to the values used in the analysis. A change in any value may or may not change the best path. A robust analysis tests the conclusions over a wide range of values to accommodate most clinical situations the practitioner is likely to encounter. If the same conclusion is reached over this wide range, its credibility increases greatly. An astute practitioner examines the range of values over which the model is tested (using sensitivity analysis) before accepting its conclusions for a patient.

If the patient's situation is well represented by a sound decision analysis and if the physician is able to tailor the utilities and other presumptions to reflect accurately the local conditions, the decision analysis provides a powerful way to improve care through probabilistic reasoning.

## SUMMARY

After years of working with all types of evidence and decision-support tools, I have concluded that an applicable and valid decision tree is among the best techniques available for evidence-based decision making. A powerful argument can be made that a decision analysis, rather than a clinical guideline or pathway, should be the gold standard for disease management. It profoundly recognizes the individual patient's values, is amenable to quantitative testing and analysis, and makes the underlying clinical reasoning blatantly obvious.

Faced with complex clinical decisions, practitioners should seek out decision analyses; if none are available, they should seek local expertise for the generation of a decision tree once all the evidence has been gathered. If no expert is available, perhaps the practitioner might take on the task of learning how to master the decision analysis (see the references for background information). The practitioner's clinical reasoning gains much for such efforts.

## REFERENCES

1. Detsky AS and others: Tutorial: how to perform a decision analysis, *Med Decis Making* 17(2):123-152, 1997.
2. Gross RA: *Making medical decisions,* Philadelphia, 1999, American College of Physicians.
3. Protheroe J and others: The impact of patients' preferences on the treatment of atrial fibrillation: observational study of patient based decision analysis, *BMJ* 320(7246):1380-1384, 2000.
4. Sox HC and others: *Medical decision making,* Stoneham, Mass, 1988, Butterworth-Heinemann.
5. Wells PS and others: Use of a clinical model for safe management of patients with suspected pulmonary embolism, *Ann Intern Med* 129(12):997-1005, 1998.

# CHAPTER 10

# Studies in Evidence-Based Decision Making

## INTRODUCTION

The preceding chapters have covered a great deal of material. This chapter is intended to assist readers in putting this new knowledge to work. For each of two of the most important types of evidence discussed—therapy and diagnosis—two cases are presented. The first case is presented in some detail, with ample commentary regarding how to approach it from an evidence-based perspective. A second "on-your-own" case is presented for the reader to solve independently, although a few hints provide guides in the right direction. A "hint" section for each on-your-own case is provided at the end of the chapter, but readers should work through the cases independently before reading the hints.

Readers considering the cases in this chapter should remember that medical evidence by nature changes rapidly. Thus the "correct" conclusion as of this writing may not be correct for all readers at all times. The important concept is that the best evidence available at the time the decision must be made is used and that sound decision-making skills are applied at all times.

The cases presented in this chapter do not necessarily "work out" perfectly. Included are examples of incomplete, inconclusive, or inconsistent evidence; scenarios in which the evidence is not quite applicable; and other phenomena that reflect realistic occurrences, not only perfect textbook cases. The hope is that after wallowing through such less-than-ideal situations, readers are better equipped to deal with such cases in practice.

Throughout the chapter, readers should adhere to the "FRAP" approach, as follows:

- *F*raming of the question
- *R*etrieval of the evidence
- *A*ppraisal of the evidence
- *P*atient application of the conclusions

These steps are presented as "tasks" in the cases to follow.

# *Questions of Treatment*

# TREATMENT OF ULCERATIVE COLITIS

Therapy Case 1

A 31-year-old man is admitted to the hospital for treatment of a severe exacerbation of ulcerative colitis. His initial treatment includes moderately high doses of corticosteroids, hydration, and dietary restrictions, with increases as tolerated. After 7 days, he continues to experience frequent diarrhea, rectal bleeding, and a weight loss of 8 pounds.

Various parameters of nutritional status are obtained and show no evidence of severe malnutrition. Although not in acute distress, he appears chronically ill and is frustrated with his lack of progress. He is not vomiting, and serial abdominal exams and radiographs do not demonstrate evidence of toxic megacolon. A gastroenterology consultation is obtained, and the consultant confirms your general plan of care, also suggesting the institution of total parenteral nutrition.

You are unfamiliar with the potential benefits and risks of total parenteral nutrition in this setting and thus decide to learn more about it before you choose to implement this recommendation.

**Task #1: Frame the dilemma as an evidence-based question.**

Is this a question of diagnosis, therapy, risk, prognosis, or some other category? In the present case, total parenteral nutrition is clearly a therapeutic intervention. The evidence to obtain is whether this course of action improves the course of patients with exacerbation of ulcerative colitis and, if so, at what expense. Before building the question, readers should recognize that the case involves an acute exacerbation and not chronic disease; a young, otherwise healthy patient; and a scenario that lacks acute or emergent findings.

Also useful is to identify the target outcomes the physician hopes the treatment can improve. In this case, contenders might include length of hospital stay, time until resolution or marked improvement of symptoms, or avoidance of colectomy. Thus the evidence-based question might resemble the following:

In acute exacerbations of ulcerative colitis in otherwise healthy patients, does total parenteral nutrition reduce length of day, time until recovery, or need for surgery?

More specifically, what are the parameters typically used to express the effectiveness of therapy? Absolute and relative risk reductions (ARRs and RRRs), from which to calculate number needed to treat (NNT) and, for the adverse effects, number needed to harm (NNH), must be sought to help determine an answer. Readers who require a refresher on the meanings of these terms are advised to refer to Chapter 3.

**Task #2: Retrieve applicable, valid, and current evidence to answer the question at hand.**

Because this question involves therapy, several resource options may be consulted for the desired evidence. Among these are the Cochrane Library, Best Evidence, and of course, MEDLINE, as follows:

- **Cochrane:** Because the search strategies discussed for therapy are designed to work with MEDLINE in particular, a search of the Cochrane Library (a much smaller resource than MEDLINE) can proceed with the use of keywords alone. I searched under the query *ulcerative colitis* and found 10 citations. A title scan identified none as applicable.
  *Time spent:* 39 seconds
- **Best Evidence:** This search found 25 citations, none of which appears applicable on a title scan.
  *Time spent:* 50 seconds
- **MEDLINE via PubMed:** In this database the formal search strategies again must be used.

  **Pass 1:** ulcerative colitis AND total parenteral nutrition AND (therap* OR random*)
  *Results:* 129 citations
  **Pass 2:** #1 AND randomized controlled trial
  *Results:* 6

  Scanning these citations by title identifies two of potential applicability. The first is titled "Enteral versus parenteral nutrition as adjunct therapy in acute ulcerative colitis"[7] and the second, "Controlled trial of intravenous hyperalimentation and total bowel rest as an adjunct to the routine therapy of acute colitis."[4]
  *Time spent:* 120 seconds

The total time spent to search and scan all three resources was less than 4 minutes.

### Task #3: Appraise the evidence for applicability and validity. What are the results?

This task is performed for the Gonzales-Huix article.[7] Following is its abstract, but practitioners should only appraise the article in its complete form:

To ascertain the role of total enteral nutrition, compared with total parenteral nutrition, as adjunct therapy to steroids in patients with severe acute ulcerative colitis, a prospective randomized trial was conducted in 42 of such patients. Inclusion criteria were the persistence of a moderate or severe attack of the disease (Truelove's index) after 48 h on full steroid treatment (prednisone 1 mg/kg/day). Patients were randomized to receive polymeric total enteral nutrition or isocaloric, isonitrogenous total parenteral nutrition as the sole nutritional support. Remission rate and need for colectomy were similar in both groups. No significant changes in anthropometric parameters were observed in either nutritional group at the end of the study. Median increase in serum albumin was 16.7% (−0.5% to +30.4%) in the enteral feeding group, and only 4.6% (−12.0% to

+13.7%) in the parenteral nutrition patients (p = 0.019). Adverse effects related to artificial nutritional support were less frequent (9% vs. 35%, p = 0.046) and milder in enterally fed patients. Postoperative infections occurred more often with parenteral nutrition (p = 0.028). These results suggest that total enteral nutrition is safe and nutritionally effective in severe attacks of ulcerative colitis. It is also cheaper and associated with fewer complications than parenteral nutrition. Total enteral nutrition should be regarded as the most suitable type of nutritional support in these patients.

## Applicability

### Does the Study Fit My Patient from a Biographic and Biologic Perspective?
Table 2 in the article shows the subjects to be of both genders, young, and with disease severity comparable to that of the patient in question. A bit fewer than half of studied subjects were in their first attack of the disease, leaving the other half of longer but unspecified disease duration. The study compared total enteral nutrition via a feeding tube to parenteral nutrition. The patient in the example was receiving oral feedings as tolerated. This discrepancy may be important, but the reader should defer judgment for now.

### Is the Outcome Inventory Sufficiently Complete for My Patient?
The study examined the achievement of mild or inactive disease maintainable with doses of prednisone lower than 30 mg per day. Severity was assessed by use of a standardized objective scale (Truelove and Witt's criteria). Treatment failure was well defined. The outcomes studied seem acceptable, although the length of stay was not reported explicitly.

The study appears reasonably applicable, with the previously stated reservations.

## Validity

**The RCB Rule** Were the subjects enrolled and assigned to their respective groups in a manner that was *R*andom, *C*oncealed, and *B*lind (RCB)? The authors state that group assignment was randomized. Whether concealment was enforced is unclear (that is, whether the persons responsible for excluding subjects from the study knew to which groups they would have been assigned had they been included), and because 38 of 82 subjects initially enrolled were excluded, this subject is a concern. Fortunately, the exclusion criteria seem objective and obvious—colonic megacolon, perforation, severe hemorrhage, obstruction, and inability to remain on nutritional support for at least 7 days. The study was *not* blinded.

Thus major potential deficiencies in the study design are identified, especially the lack of blinding. The only way to "forgive" this particular deficiency is if the outcome criteria are substantially bullet proof against subjective assessment. The Truelove criteria used are not delineated explicitly in the paper, leaving this burden to the reader—no small task, given the 1955 publication date of the reference for this disease severity scale. Fortunately, a standard gastroenterology textbook[5] describes them as follows:

- *Mild*—less than four stools daily, with or without blood, with no systemic disturbance and a normal erythrocyte sedimentation rate (ESR)
- *Moderate*—more than four stools daily but with minimal systemic disturbance
- *Severe*—more than six stools daily, with blood, with evidence of systemic disturbance as shown by fever, tachycardia, anemia, or an ESR of more than 30

Given the objective nature of most of these criteria, the lack of blinding may not be fatal to the validity of the study.

**The Follow-Through Rule** All the subjects who entered the study were followed to its conclusion in their original groups; one from each group left the study because of severe complications of the disease. An intention-to-treat analysis confirmed that this dropout rate was not important to the study's conclusions; even if the two subjects had remained in the study, its conclusions would not have changed.

At this point the study is deemed to be of acceptable if not optimal primary validity. The secondary validity criteria next are consulted.

**Comparable Groups** The paper provides a table confirming that the groups were comparable, other than regarding the nutritional intervention. Age, severity score, laboratory results, and demographics were compared explicitly.

As for comparable treatment throughout the study, the paper confirms that all patients received similar doses of oral and rectal steroids, as well as supportive therapy "when necessary." The reader is left to assume that supportive measures (transfusion, albumin, fluids) were administered in an unbiased fashion but to wonder whether differences may have occurred, and whether these differences could have biased the outcomes. Such bias seems unlikely, but some concern still remains.

**Complications of Total Parenteral Nutrition** The study resulted in a 24% absolute risk (AR; 35% versus 9%) for complications in the total parenteral nutrition group, compared with the enteral group. Of these complications, 2 of 20 (10%) proved serious—subclavian thrombosis and sepsis.

**Validity Summary** This study is judged to be of flawed validity primarily due to the absence of blinding, uncertain concealment, and uncertainty about whether overall management between the two groups was entirely comparable. As noted, none of these concerns was deemed fatal due to offsetting assumptions and adherence to objective outcome criteria. Nonetheless, the study's validity is considered less than ideal.

**The Results** Eight of 20 (60%) experimental (parenteral) group subjects and 12 of 22 (46%) control group subjects failed to achieve remission. (Phrasing the results in terms of bad outcomes is useful because it enables the use of risk reduction as the outcome number.) Serious harm occurred in 9% of the experimental group and in 0% of the control group. Thus the ARR for "unremitting disease" was 14% [95% CI = −15% to 44%, *CI* being the *confidence interval*]. The AR for harm from parenteral nutrition was 10% [95% CI = −3% to 23%].

These results are interpreted to mean that the study failed to demonstrate a statistically significant difference in remission rates in subjects treated with parenteral nutrition, compared with those treated with enteral nutrition. Because of the small group sizes, the observed differences are too small to use to draw any conclusions. (The CIs for ARR included 0% by quite a large margin.)

> *Important:* The study did not prove that *no* difference existed; it simply *failed* to demonstrate that a difference *did* exist. That is, a study 10 times its size yielding the *exact same ARR of 14%* would have a CI of 5% to 24%, making it statistically significant. (This calculation is done with a computer program; the reader is not expected to have performed this last projection).

What about the harm? The CIs around the 10% AR showed lack of statistical significance, even though a trend toward significance did exist. (The CI did include 0, but not by much, with most of the interval lying on the side of true harm). This observation means that although the CI of −3% to 23% was not significant, the range is "asymmetric enough" on the greater-than-zero side for the trend to raise concerns (especially in the absence of improvement). Added to the fact that the complications in question could not have occurred plausibly in the control group (by use of clinical knowledge about subclavian thrombosis and catheter sepsis), and the potential for harm should be taken quite seriously.

### Task #4: Given the risks and improvements shown by the evidence for this treatment, should you treat the patient?

The previous discussion concluded that the evidence is applicable and of acceptable if not of perfect validity but that it fails to demonstrate benefit even though the study was small; it demonstrates possible harm. In this context a practitioner may be hard pressed to imagine any set of values or preferences on the patient's part that would warrant treatment with parenteral nutrition to hasten remission for the exacerbation of ulcerative colitis. As an aside, however, a practitioner might recommend this treatment for severe and progressive malnutrition—but not to induce disease remission.

### Summary

This case illustrates that way in which an evidence-based decision making (EBDM) approach can be used for therapy questions. Elements of the search strategy prove useful and necessary; appraisal of validity and applicability reveals good correlation; statistical significance issues become important; and clinical judgment enters the picture. Readers can use this experience to practice EBDM on their own.

## TREATMENT OF ACUTE BRONCHITIS

> *Therapy Case 2 (On Your Own)*
>
> Your busy patient describes 5 days of nasal congestion and a cough that was nonproductive initially but in the past 3 days has produced moderate amounts of thick yellow sputum with no blood. He has not experienced fever, chills, chest pain, dyspnea, stiff neck, or other relevant symptoms, but the cough is interfering with his sleep and work productivity. He is not a smoker, and his medical history is negative for heart, lung, immune, and other serious disease. A physical exam is normal, specifically negative for signs of pulmonary consolidation, cardiac dysfunction, or hypoxemia. Assume that no extraneous history or findings are present.
>
> After reading about bronchitis on the Internet, the patient reports that he seems to have bronchitis and requests that you prescribe an antibiotic. Although you have faced this situation countless times, the patient's apparent challenge prompts you to arm yourself with the best evidence before helping him to make a decision.

**Task #1: Frame the dilemma as an evidence-based question.**
**Task #2: Retrieve applicable, valid, and current evidence to answer the question at hand.**
**Task #3: Appraise the evidence for applicability and validity. What are the results?**
**Task #4: Given the risks and improvements shown by the evidence for this treatment, should you treat this patient?**

Readers should feel free to read the hints provided at the end of this chapter but are advised to do so *after* working through the problem independently.

## PULMONARY EMBOLUS IN A NEUROLOGICALLY IMPAIRED PATIENT

> *Diagnosis Case 1*
>
> A colleague in the rehabilitation department requests your advice on a patient who is paraplegic from a spinal cord injury resulting from a motorcycle crash and who currently is undergoing rehabilitation. This

24-year-old man developed an episode of diaphoresis and mild shortness of breath that lasted several hours late the previous day. Today he feels better but remains mildly dyspneic in bed, with a respiratory rate of 16.

The rehabilitation staff obtained Doppler studies of his legs, and they were negative. His chest radiograph showed bibasilar infiltrates consistent with atelectasis. His oxygen saturation was 88%. A blood test for d-dimer was obtained and returned negative. A lung scan was attempted, but due to the presence of orthopedic devices around the neck and chest and difficulty with transfer, it was technically suboptimal; the scan did show matched ventilation and perfusion defects in the lower lung fields.

The referring physician requests your help in deciding what to do next. All parties accept that treatment with anticoagulation for pulmonary embolism has an action threshold (AT) of about 5%. (That is, its improvements outweigh its risks if the clinical likelihood of the disease is above this level.)

### Task #1: Frame the dilemma as an evidence-based question.

This complex situation is such that even the framing of a question about the diagnostic tests (ultrasound, lung scan, d-dimer) is not a trivial task. In addition, an evidence-based pretest disease likelihood estimate must be determined based on clinical data.[12] The following question forms the substrate for the decision (that is, the pretest estimate of the disease):

What is the probability of pulmonary embolus in high-risk patients presenting with acute dyspnea?

In this case a pretest estimate of the likelihood of pulmonary embolus in this clinical context is judged to be approximately 40%.* Next, the already-known Doppler results must be applied to that figure. From a d-dimer perspective, these figures are all considered "pretest." *Pretest* refers to the likelihood of the use of all information available *before the test in question is performed.*

The discussion now turns to the question that must be framed for the diagnostic tests themselves. Ultimately, most practitioners would like to know likelihood ratios (LRs); because LRs are calculated from sensitivity and specificity, the questions to answer include the following:

What are the sensitivity and specificity of venous Doppler ultrasound, lung scan, and d-dimer for pulmonary embolus?

This question manages to ask three pieces of information for one scenario.

---

*This pretest estimate is not simply a guess; it was derived by a review of the evidence found in the articles about the tests themselves. That is, the studies about the Doppler ultrasound and d-dimer included populations similar to that of the patient in the example, and the risks that could be used as a starting point. In addition, the article cited looked at the accuracy of clinical assessment directly in stating a diagnosis of pulmonary embolus and provided specific risk data. Thus the term *pretest estimate* may not do justice to the accuracy in this scenario; the 40% figure is quite accurate as a starting point.

**Task #2: Retrieve applicable, valid, and current evidence to answer the question at hand. What are the results?**

The user might proceed directly to MEDLINE for these focused bits of evidence, starting with Doppler studies. (Remember: Cochrane is for therapy evidence only. Where else might a user begin other than with MEDLINE?)

> **Pass 1:** pulmonary embolism AND venous Doppler AND (diagnos* OR sens*)
> *Results:* 181 citations
> **Pass 2:** #1 AND sensitivity AND specificity
> *Results:* 38 citations

The pass 2 yield of 38 is a manageable number. Not surprisingly, the evidence focused on the Doppler technique for *deep vein thrombosis*, not for pulmonary embolus.[8] None of the retrieved articles addressed that issue specifically; title scanning was not promising. At this time, the user may consider reassessing the search strategy.*

The use of the phrase *venous Doppler* as a key term may draw the attention of the astute searcher because in the initial title review the term *ultrasound* was used far more frequently. The medical subject heading (MeSH) and phrase mapping features may not have been activated in this instance. Substituting the phrase *venous ultraso** (to catch any articles that include the term *ultrasonography,* as well) produces a set of different results.

> **Pass 1:** pulmonary embolism AND venous ultraso* AND (diagnos* OR sens*)
> *Results:* 384 citations (compared with 181 on the initial pass 1)
> **Pass 2:** #1 AND sensitivity AND specificity
> *Results:* 79 (compared with 38 in the initial pass 2)

This time the title scan identified several promising citations, including two that appear highly applicable.[13-14]

The sample search got a bit cumbersome. Suppose a MEDLINE search had been deferred, replaced with an initial search of Best Evidence. In this case, a search for the phrase *pulmonary embolism* alone found a neatly compiled critical appraisal of the Turkstra[13] article, commentary and all.[1] The lesson in this case is to begin searching with trusted, preappraised data repositories and proceed to MEDLINE only as a double-check for more recent evidence or if the initial search results are unconvincing.

For the d-dimer test the search proceeds to Best Evidence directly. Searching for the term *d-dimer* alone (because the fancy filters and strategies are in-

---

*This type of improvisational refinement of search strategies is commonplace. When the search results are surprising or disappointing, the medical subject heading (MeSH) setting should be verified; typographic errors, if any, located; and rephrasing of the keywords considered.

tended only for MEDLINE) yields 15 citations, including one highly relevant study[6] that stratifies patients by clinical risk levels.

### Task #3: Appraise the evidence for applicability and validity. What are the results?

From the abstract scan, the Turkstra[13] article seemed to be the most rigorous review, so this discussion focuses on that citation. The other studies were done in an ambulatory environment,[3] a postoperative setting,[9] or were conspicuously less methodologically rigorous.

Applying the diagnosis criteria for applicability (patient similarity, disease spectrum, practicality of doing the tests locally) and validity (independent gold standard applied universally, blinding where appropriate, test described fully), a judgment is made that this article is sufficiently suitable to proceed.

The negative LR [LR− = (1 − sensitivity) ÷ specificity] of venous ultrasound for pulmonary embolism based on this evidence is as follows:

$$LR- = \frac{(1 - 0.29)}{0.97} = 0.73 \text{ (not very robust)}$$

The focus turns now to the d-dimer test. Readers should assume that the Ginsberg[6] article meets the required validity criteria because it was approved by the editorial board of *ACP Journal Club* (an assumption not necessarily proper for all journals). Further reading would place the patient in the example in the nondiagnostic lung scan category; therefore the figure of 0.36 (obtained from the Ginsberg[6] article) is most appropriate as the negative LR of d-dimer (specifically in patients with nondiagnostic lung scans). Its positive LR is 2.2.

## Pretest Likelihood

The pretest estimate is not a simple guess; it is derived by a review of the evidence in the articles previously stated as relevant to the case at hand. That is, the studies about the Doppler ultrasound and d-dimer include populations similar to that of the patient in question, and their risk for pulmonary embolus thus can be used as a starting point. Furthermore, during the title scan, a citation highly relevant to pretest risk is located[14] by direct reference from the Ginsberg[6] article (and in the same issue!); this finding adds further support to the pretest estimate. From these sources, assumptions are made that the patient is high risk (78% risk) and that a nondiagnostic lung scan lowers this risk to 47%,[6] or in other words, odds of 0.89 (47% ÷ 53%).

### Task #4: Given the likelihood ratios shown by the evidence, the pretest probability estimate, and the available treatment options, would performing this test help the patient?

The previous discussion noted that the patient would receive treatment if the probability of pulmonary embolism were greater than 5% (this being the AT), and that the pretest estimate for high-risk patients with nondiagnostic lung scans was around 47% (odds of 0.89). Given the negative LR of venous ultrasound (0.73), the pretest estimate before the performance of a d-dimer is as follows:

$$\text{Posttest odds} = \text{pretest odds} \times LR$$

$$= 0.89 \times 0.73 = 0.65, \text{or } 39\%$$

where *LR* is the likelihood ratio.

Note how LRs can be used in sequence to generate an ongoing set of disease likelihoods (clinical odds × lung scan LR × ultrasound LR, etc.); the posttest probability after each test becomes the new "pretest" estimate for the subsequent test. This technique is sound as long as the tests in question measure biologically independent aspects of the disease, which in this case they seem to do.

Finally, a "new" pretest estimate is established for d-dimer, in this sequence: 39%, or odds of 0.65. Applying the negative LR for d-dimer produces the following result:

$$\text{Posttest odds} = \text{pretest odds} \times LR-$$

$$= 0.65 \times 0.36 = 0.23, \text{or } 19\%$$

where $LR-$ is the negative likelihood ratio. For a positive d-dimer result the calculation is as follows:

$$\text{Posttest odds} = \text{pretest odds} \times LR+$$

$$= 0.65 \times 2.2 = 1.43, \text{or } 59\%$$

where $LR+$ is the positive likelihood ratio.

## Interpreting the Analysis

Where does this information leave the case? Because a diagnostic probability of even 5% has been established to warrant treatment, performance of a test that at best would decrease the suspicion of disease no lower than 19% does not seem to be very useful. Treatment would be the choice if the test were negative and, of course, if it were positive. Thus a d-dimer in this case may not be worth the trouble. In the patient in question, the definitive test—pulmonary angiography—probably is indicated. If the test is negative, the patient is spared the risk of many months of anticoagulation; if it turns up positive, the test provides assurance that the risk is justified by the strong benefits of such treatment when pulmonary embolism is present.

## Summary

This example is a complex diagnostic situation with many factors to consider. It involves somewhat ambiguous clinical factors, several "serial" diagnostic tests, and a gold-standard test (angiography) that is somewhat invasive and a bit risky. Most cases are far less onerous. Readers who were able to follow the reasoning and arithmetic in this case truly have mastered the necessary concepts. If not, a second reading of this material by section may prove helpful; broken down into its various components, the example is not as difficult as it may seem when taken as a whole. The "on-your-own" case that follows is much easier to follow and may prove quite useful in practice.

## CHEST X-RAY FOR ACUTE COUGH

*Diagnosis Case 2 (On Your Own)*

A senior colleague in your office (who oversees your managed-care contracts) has suggested tactfully that you may be ordering far more chest x-rays to exclude pneumonia on your managed-care population than the rest of the group. She claims that with good clinical judgment, you could order fewer radiographs without compromising the quality of care. You are eager to learn from her experience, so you inquire as to which findings or rules she uses to decide when to obtain a film.

After some deliberation, she states that in otherwise uncompromised patients, if they have no significant fever (less than 38° C) she rarely orders an x-ray; if the exam shows no signs of consolidation (rales, dullness) she does not order an x-ray, but if the respiratory rate is more than 18 or so, she generally will order x-rays. These guidelines sound reasonable to you, but you wonder about their basis in evidence.

**Task #1: Frame the dilemma as an evidence-based question.**

Remember that physical exam findings and history items can be considered diagnostic tests.

**Task #2: Retrieve applicable, valid, and current evidence to answer the question at hand.**

**Task #3: Appraise the evidence for applicability and validity. What are the results?**

As always, both sensitivity and specificity should be sought to calculate LRs.

**Task #4: Given the evidence, what guidelines would you use to determine when an x-ray is warranted?**

You may assume that pneumonia is present in around 5% of outpatients with acute cough.[10-11] This figure is the pretest probability.

## Summary

For those readers who see such patients, this case exemplifies the situation in which the practitioner might not perform such a complete EBDM analysis for each individual patient, but rather do so once to form a practice "strategy" that can be applied generally in practice.

# *Hints and Solutions to 'On-Your-Own' Cases*

## ACUTE BRONCHITIS

**Task #1: Frame the dilemma as an evidence-based question.**

In uncomplicated patients with symptoms of acute bronchitis, do antibiotics shorten the duration of symptoms? What is the probability of complications resulting from such treatment?

**Task #2: Retrieve applicable, valid, and current evidence to answer the question at hand.**

A wise strategy is to search under the term *acute bronchitis* in Cochrane Library and Best Evidence. For MEDLINE, the phrase *acute bronchitis AND (random\* OR therap\*)* should be used, followed by *#1 AND randomized controlled trial*. The latter search should narrow the findings down to approximately 50 to 60 articles. Many are head-to-head comparisons of two antibiotics, of interest only if the efficacy of *any* antibiotic is accepted. This problem makes the evidence tricky to interpret.

For instance, if the searcher were a pharmaceutical company with a new antibiotic, comparison of the new drug with one or two of the most widely used antibiotics for this condition may prove useful. If the drug in question proved equally effective, the pharmaceutical company could join the fray with its new product to compete with existing products already on the market. However, if neither drug proved effective, such a study would not be of value other than for business purposes.

In such a situation, the Cochrane-type citation can be of great use.[2] That database makes an active effort to retrieve negative as well as positive studies.

**Task #3: Appraise the evidence for applicability and validity. What are the results?**

*For applicability:* Does the study fit the patient in question from a biographic and biologic perspective? The practitioner must pay attention to the duration of illness at the time of presentation and the diagnostic criteria. Are all the outcomes of interest to this situation included in the studies? Are the antibiotics used the same as, or similar to, the ones the practitioner would select?

*For validity:* Was the study RCB? If blinding was not a criterion, are the outcome criteria vulnerable to subjective bias? Was follow-through complete and sufficient in length, and were initial group assignments maintained? Were the groups comparable at the outset and treated identically, other than for the study agent?

If Cochrane Library or Best Evidence reviews are being used, the practitioner can assume that this was done already.

*The results:* The goal is to try to phrase the results as risk reduction; therefore if symptom duration reduction of 24 hours is the criterion for a clinically significant effect, for example, what percentage of subjects achieved this benchmark in each group? If possible, the results can be described as an ARR, then as an NNT (100/ARR), with a similar process used for side effects, if any, to obtain an NNH.

**Task #4: Given the risks and improvements shown by the evidence for this treatment, should you treat this patient?**

Is the ratio of the harm (impact $\times$ frequency) to clinical improvement (impact $\times$ frequency) less than 1 (the AT)? If not, the practitioner would advise against treatment. If this ratio is very close to 1, treatment still may not be indicated because issues of community antibiotic resistance and cost might offset any trivial gain for this patient.

The best evidence suggests that modest benefit, if any, is derived; that many of the underlying studies are flawed; and that the harm, although small, probably mitigates any existing improvement. Adding to those facts are the general risk of community antibiotic resistance and cost to use this therapy routinely, and treatment with antibiotic seems like an action generally to be avoided in this context.

How might the practitioner decline the patient's request while still addressing his need for "intervention"? I have found that in addition to symptomatic measures, a statement such as the following goes a long way:

> *"Try this (symptomatic) treatment for 3 days; if you do not notice any improvement at that point, we can reassess the risks and benefits of antibiotics by phone."*

Most patients feel better and for those who do not, a clinical reassessment may well be appropriate at any rate. Such a statement leaves the door open to the possibility of antibiotics and acknowledges the legitimacy of the patient's request.

## DIAGNOSIS: PNEUMONIA

**Task #1: Frame the dilemma as an evidence-based question.**

The practitioner asks, as a diagnostic question, what the LRs are for various office-based exam findings or history items. Based on the results of these "tests," decisions are made regarding which patients should receive chest x-rays. Physical findings are no different from other diagnostic tests, other than that they are essentially free of risk and cost (above that of the visit).

**Task #2: Retrieve applicable, valid, and current evidence to answer the question at hand.**

The search should begin with Best Evidence, after which MEDLINE should be considered. For the former database, key terms such as *pneumonia* and *physical examination* serve as good starting points. For MEDLINE, the two-pass search strategy should be used.

**Pass 1:** pneumonia and "physical examination" AND (diagnos* OR sens*)
**Pass 2:** #1 AND sensitivity AND specificity

Pass 2 sometimes filters out articles of interest inadvertently; unless the number of citations in pass 1 is very high, the user may find that scanning the titles before automatically proceeding to pass 2 is worthwhile. This case provides a good illustration of this inadvertent-filtering phenomenon.

### Task #3: Appraise the evidence for applicability and validity. What are the results?

The ideal evidence is a systematic review, in which the validity criteria are preappraised. Lacking that, the usual criteria must be used—independent blind comparison with a gold standard, appropriate patient spectrum, etc. In terms of applicability the practitioner can do well to remember that these are community-based outpatients.

My citation of choice for this dilemma was that of Metlay and colleagues in the 1997 *Journal of the American Medical Association.*[11] The results of interest are found in the tables. For example, the LRs (positive, negative) for some of the findings in this case are as follows:

- Fever (1.4 to 4.4, 0.58 to 0.78)
- Rales (1.7 to 2.7, 0.62 to 0.87)
- Dullness (2.2 to 4.3, 0.79 to 0.93)
- Respiratory rate more than 20 (1.2 and 0.66)

### Task #4: Given the evidence, what guidelines would you use to determine when an x-ray is warranted?

*Hint:* The rules selected enable the practitioner to predict how many x-rays to obtain to find one case of pneumonia. Only the practitioner can determine the acceptable percentage. Would two normal radiographs for every case of pneumonia be tolerable? Would 100? The cost would be in both dollars and in occasional incidental findings, which create unnecessary anxiety, follow-up studies, and so forth.

To go out on a limb a bit, my personal judgment (based on the importance of immediate diagnosis of pneumonia versus the direct and indirect costs of an x-ray) is that a positive-to-negative rate in the range of 5:1 would be excellent; even 10:1 might be suitable. The patients who are "missed" by the practitioner's not being more "liberal" in the ordering pattern usually can be recaptured by reporting back for persistent or worsening symptoms.

Therefore by use of this criteria, any rule that would get the practitioner from the pretest likelihood of 5% (odds of 0.05) to a posttest likelihood of 10% to 20% (odds of 0.11 to 0.25), which is the tolerance level for the yield of chest x-rays, would be useful. The likelihood ratio for a test required to achieve a 10:1 normal-to-abnormal x-ray ratio thus would be calculated as follows:

$$\text{Posttest odds} = \text{pretest odds} \times \text{LR+}$$

$$11 = 0.05 \times \text{LR+}$$

$$\text{LR+} = 2.2$$

For a 5:1 "success rate" the positive LR would be 5. The practitioner then must determine whether any of the prediction rules in the previously located citations have a positive LR of 2.2 or higher.

## Summary

A final comment on this scenario is that a substantial value judgment remains in terms of how willing the practitioner would be to accept a given ratio of normal-to-abnormal chest films. One might wonder whether this subjectivity degrades the value of performing such a quantitative analysis in the face of such variability over how to apply it. In fact a practitioner's knowing how the clinical practice patterns affect the outcomes is the key to good decision making. Although uncertainty about any given patient persists, the practitioner now has the tools necessary to decide how much uncertainty is acceptable and how to practice to reach those value-driven goals.

This approach can be compared to that of the senior colleague who initially questioned the exam-ordering practices, which were essentially based on experience. She had no idea what her precise rules for making the decision really were, what effect that uncertainty had on her diagnostic accuracy, and certainly no means of knowing whether her practices were acceptable or unacceptable by any standard because she could not predict their impact on her patients.

## REFERENCES

1. Abstract for 'Compression ultrasonography had limited value for detecting pulmonary embolism,' *ACP J Club* 127:75, 1997.
2. Becker L and others: Antibiotics for acute bronchitis (Cochrane review). In *The Cochrane Library,* issue 2, Oxford, 2000, Update Software.
3. Daniel KR, Jackson RE, Kline JA: Utility of lower extremity venous ultrasound scanning in the diagnosis and exclusion of pulmonary embolism in outpatients, *Ann Emerg Med* 35(6):547-554, 2000.
4. Dickinson RJ and others: Controlled trial of intravenous hyperalimentation and total bowel rest as an adjunct to the routine therapy of acute colitis, *Gastroenterology* 79(6):1199-1204, 1980.
5. Feldman: *Sleisenger & Fordtran's gastrointestinal and liver disease,* ed 6, Philadelphia, 1998, WB Saunders.
6. Ginsberg JS and others: Sensitivity and specificity of a rapid whole-blood assay for d-dimer in the diagnosis of pulmonary embolism, *Ann Intern Med* 129:1006-1011, 1998.
7. Gonzalez-Huix F and others: Enteral versus parenteral nutrition as adjunct therapy in acute ulcerative colitis, *Am J Gastroenterol* 88(2):227-232, 1993.
8. Kearon C, Ginsberg JS, Hirsh J: The role of venous ultrasonography in the diagnosis of suspected deep venous thrombosis and pulmonary embolism, *Ann Intern Med* 129(12):1044-1049, 1998.
9. Killewich LA, Nunnelee JD, Auer AI: Value of lower extremity venous duplex examination in the diagnosis of pulmonary embolism, *J Vasc Surg* 17(5):934-938, 1993 [discussion 938-939].
10. Metlay JP and others: National trends in the management of acute cough by primary care physicians, *J Gen Intern Med* 12(suppl):77, 1997.
11. Metlay JP and others: Does this patient have community-acquired pneumonia?: diagnosing pneumonia by history and physical examination, *JAMA* 278(17):1440-1445, 1997.
12. Miniati M and others: Accuracy of clinical assessment in the diagnosis of pulmonary embolism, *Am J Respir Crit Care Med* 159(3):864-871, 1999.
13. Turkstra F and others: Diagnostic utility of ultrasonography of leg veins in patients suspected of having pulmonary embolism, *Ann Intern Med* 126(10):775-781, 1997.
14. Wells PS and others: Use of a clinical model for safe management of patients with suspected pulmonary embolism, *Ann Intern Med* 129(12):997-1005, 1998.

## Summary of Strategies

### Therapy

| | |
|---|---|
| **Master Evidence Question** | In patients like mine, what are the frequencies of the side effects and disease outcome improvements in treated subjects, compared with those who did not receive the treatment?<br>(For results reported as means or scalar scores only, select a degree of improvement you consider clinically significant and attempt to derive frequencies for that degree of change.) |
| **Searching\*** | Cochrane, Best Evidence, and other preappraised sources should be consulted before MEDLINE.<br>For MEDLINE the following search strategy is recommended:<br><br>**Pass 1:** keywords AND (random\* OR therap\*)<br>**Pass 2:** #1 AND (randomized controlled trial) |
| **Applicability** | Does the evidence demonstrate a biologic, clinical, and demographic fit with my patient? Are outcomes of interest all included? |
| **Validity** | *RCB:* Was the study randomized, concealed (not always reported), and blind (unless all outcomes are bulletproof to lack of blinding)?<br>*Follow-through:* Was the study complete and sufficiently long? Were the original study group assignments maintained (intention-to-treat analysis)?<br>*Comparable groups:* Were the study groups well matched and treated comparably, other than for the treatment in question? |
| **Results** | Absolute risk reduction (ARR) = CER − EER<br>Number needed to treat (NNT) = 1 ÷ ARR<br>Number needed to harm (NNH) = 1 ÷ absolute risk of complication<br>Relative risk (RR) = EER ÷ CER |
| **Master Decision Question** | Is this treatment worth recommending? How does it compare to the alternatives?<br><br>Impact = importance of outcome (good or bad) on 0-to-1 scale<br>Harm = frequency × impact for bad outcomes (side effects)<br>Improvement = frequency × impact for good outcomes (disease improvements)<br>Action threshold (AT)† = harm ÷ improvement<br><br>*After all appropriate testing is complete, if . . .*<br>AT > 1, do not treat; AT < 1 treat. (Lower is better.) |

*CER,* Control event rate; *EER,* experimental event rate.

\*Search strategies presume direct MEDLINE access; asterisk is wild card; all fields should be searched; #1 refers to the pass 1 search in the history queue.

†AT requires assessment of patient impact estimates.

## Diagnosis

| | |
|---|---|
| **Master Evidence Question** | In patients representative of mine, what are the sensitivity and specificity of this test for this disease? |
| **Searching** | Best Evidence and other preappraised sources should be consulted before MEDLINE. For MEDLINE the following search strategy is recommended: |
| | **Pass 1:** keywords AND diagnos* OR sens* |
| | **Pass 2:** #1 AND sensitivity AND specificity |
| **Applicability** | Are the patients like mine? |
| | Does the disease "gamut" studied include my patient's disease profile? |
| | Can the test be performed comparably and practically in my locale? |
| **Validity** | Was the test blindly measured against a biologically independent gold standard that was applied uniformly? |
| | Is the testing methodology fully disclosed? |
| | Was the patient population representative of the actual population in which I would use the test? |
| **Results** | Positive likelihood ratio (LR+) = sensitivity ÷ (1 − specificity) |
| | Negative likelihood ratio (LR−) = (1 − sensitivity) ÷ specificity |
| **Master Decision Question** | Given the pretest likelihood estimate, would the results of this test move this estimate across the action threshold (AT)? |
| | If so, testing is recommended; if not, either treatment or observation is recommended, depending on the pretest estimate and AT (see Therapy box). |
| | Odds = probability ÷ (1 − probability) |
| | Posttest odds = pretest odds × LR |
| | Probability = odds ÷ (1 + odds) |

## Risk

| | |
|---|---|
| **Master Evidence Question** | Do subjects exposed to risk have a higher incidence of outcome, compared with individuals not exposed? |
| **Searching** | Best Evidence and other preappraised sources should be consulted before MEDLINE. For MEDLINE the following search strategy is recommended:<br><br>**Pass 1:** risk words AND outcome words AND (risk OR odds ratio)<br>**Pass 2:** #1 AND (cohort OR case control) |
| **Applicability** | Are the patients like mine?<br>Are the duration and intensity of exposure similar to that of my patient?<br>Is my patient's environment equally free of potential contaminating variables or exposures? |
| **Validity** | Are the groups similar except for disease status?<br>Were the groups selected from a predefined population of interest?<br>Were risk and disease status measured identically?<br>Was the duration of exposure adequate and similar?<br>Is a dose-response effect present? |
| **Results** | Relative risk (RR) = (EER − CER) ÷ CER<br>Odds ratio (case-control) = odds of exposure in affected population ÷ odds of exposure in unaffected population |
| **Master Decision Question** | Does the reduction in consequences warrant the burden of removing or reducing the exposure?<br>RRR or odds ratio should be used. |

*CER,* Control group event rate as probability (0-to-1 scale); *EER,* exposed group event rate as probability.

## Prognosis

| | |
|---|---|
| **Master Evidence Question** | What are the likelihoods and time distributions of the anticipated disease outcomes? |
| **Searching** | Best Evidence and other preappraised sources should be consulted before MEDLINE. For MEDLINE the following search strategy is recommended:<br><br>**Pass 1:** index terms AND (incidence OR prognos*)<br>**Pass 2:** #1 AND (cohort* OR follow-up) |
| **Applicability** | Are the patients like mine, including stage of disease?<br>Are all prognostic factors of importance considered? |
| **Validity** | Is the cohort well described and generally at a consistent stage in the progression of the disease?<br>Were the outcomes objectively measured and appraised comparably for all patients? If outcomes were open to subjective interpretation, were the researchers blinded as to each subject's history?<br>Was follow-up of the study group long enough and thoroughly performed?<br>Were other important factors that might affect outcomes accounted for? |
| **Results** | Probabilities of outcomes at appropriate points in time; median survival; probability-versus-time graphs |
| **Master Decision Question** | Does awareness of the likelihoods of the various outcomes over time help my patient make important life decisions? |

## Overviews

| | |
|---|---|
| **Master Evidence Question** | What is the conclusion, based on a thorough systematic review of current, valid, and applicable evidence? |
| **Searching** | Best Evidence, Cochrane, and other preappraised sources should be consulted for therapy before MEDLINE.<br>For MEDLINE the standard two-pass approach is recommended, as follows:<br><br>**Pass 1:** Determine specific evidence type (that is, treatment, prognosis, and so forth) and use the pass 1 strategy that corresponds to that category of evidence.<br>**Pass 2:** #1 AND (systematic review OR meta*) |
| **Applicability** | Use standard, category-specific criteria. |
| **Validity** | Are the search strategy and evidence resources explicitly described?<br>Are the criteria for inclusion of a research article clearly delineated, and do they meet accepted standards of critical appraisal?<br>Meta-analysis: Is the analysis weighted for study size?<br>Does it contain an appropriate statistical common denominator for all studies? |
| **Results** | Category-dependent value; often an RR, odds ratio, or LR |
| **Master Decision Question** | The question depends on the category of evidence. A suitable review with definitive conclusions is among the most powerful types of evidence available. |

*LR,* Likelihood ratio; *RR,* relative risk.

## Guidelines

| | |
|---|---|
| **Master Evidence Question** | Is this guideline based on suitable evidence, sound logic, and appropriate opinions, and is it feasible in my setting? |
| **Searching** | Specific guideline resources (for example, www.guideline.gov) should be consulted before MEDLINE.<br>For MEDLINE the following search strategy is recommended:<br><br>**Pass 1:** keywords AND (guideline OR pathway)<br>**Pass 2:** #1 AND practice guideline |
| **Applicability** | This criterion is content specific. |
| **Validity** | Are embedded value judgments present and acceptable?<br>Does the guideline address a real problem in my setting?<br>Is the flow logical and complete?<br>Is the guideline locally appropriate?<br>Is it based on sound evidence, per systematic review criteria?<br>Was the guideline prospectively validated in a separate trial? |
| **Master Decision Question** | Will using this guideline improve patient care or improve efficiency without diminishing the quality of patient care? |

## Decision Analysis

| | |
|---|---|
| **Master Evidence Question** | Does this decision analysis identify an optimal management sequence, based on sound evidence, reasonable logic, and sensible utilities? |
| **Searching** | The usual MEDLINE category-specific citations should be consulted, and/or the following two-pass search strategy should be performed:<br><br>**Pass 1:** keywords AND decision AND analy*<br>**Pass 2:** #1 AND utility |
| **Applicability** | This criterion is content specific; utilities should be acceptable. |
| **Validity** | Does the evidence used in the analysis meet the customary validity criteria for its category?<br>Is the decision logic rational and complete?<br>Are evidence or utility "soft spots" dealt with by use of appropriate sensitivity analysis?<br>Has the analysis been validated in a prospective study (uncommon)? |
| **Results** | Optimal management path, as described in the chapter |
| **Master Decision Question** | Will using this analysis improve patient care?<br>This question is often unanswerable definitively, but a sound decision analysis may provide the best evidence available. |

# Epilog

This journey through the world of evidence-based decision making (EBDM) has touched many aspects of how we, as physicians, help patients make important choices. A useful closing may be a discussion of just how readers might implement their newly acquired knowledge and skills.

Neither I nor any colleagues I have worked with perform a formal evidence search, appraisal, and decision analysis for every patient we see. Particularly unusual, complex, or serious cases exist in which this formal process is indeed carried out in much the same way presented in this book, but such cases represent a minority of patient encounters.

How, then, can readers put this material to work realistically? Following are some suggestions based on my experience:

1. At your leisure, begin by identifying the three most common problems in your specialty. These problems may seem trivial, but give this exercise a try. For each one, delineate the diagnostic and therapeutic options and choices. Then perform a full FRAP analysis (*f*rame the question, *r*etrieve the evidence, *a*ppraise the evidence, and apply it to *p*atient care) on each item identified.

   The goal of this exercise is to develop a best–evidence-based *strategy* to approach the identified problem. For example, when you next see a case of pharyngitis, you will know the three most likely pathogens, along with their percent occurrences; in addition, you will know the likelihood ratios of throat cultures for streptococcus and the harm and improvements from the available treatments. Variations on a patient-by-patient basis always are necessary, but the core evidence will be at your fingertips. You need not repeat this lengthy analysis for every patient with a sore throat once you have done it for the general approach to sore throat care.

2. The next time your usual medical journal arrives, find an article of relevance and perform a critical appraisal of it. Judge its validity and applicability to your practice; try to choose articles of different evidence types. Soon you will begin to realize that a wide variation exists in the quality of the research on which your practice is based. Become selective but not cynical. (Remember that perfect research is like the holy grail!)

3. Practice your evidence searching skills often and with real questions that arise in your practice. The logistics of evidence location are manageable but take time to acquire. The guides provided in this book can be great time savers, but become creative when the results are not what you expect. Once you become confident in finding evidence, you will be more likely to use it. In addition, do not overlook the increasing number of preappraised evidence resources available in many specialties.

4. Do not become discouraged. You may take a year or more to become a consistent evidence user. Once you get the knack for finding the right kind of evidence, you will find yourself dissatisfied with glib or anecdotal answers to important questions.
5. Remember that you are doing this analysis for your patients, not only for yourself.

We are on the verge of a medical information explosion like none we have ever experienced. Stem cell research, gene therapy, and certainly many other ideas that are inconceivable today are bound to revolutionize our profession. You can watch it happen and quickly become overwhelmed by the growing volumes of information, or you can use this information explosion efficiently and selectively by applying the tools of EBDM. Just-in-time learning is bound to replace just-in-case learning by practical necessity, if nothing else. Although background knowledge will always remain important, it will represent a progressively smaller proportion of what we need to know to practice great medicine.

Welcome to the word of EBDM believers. Your recognition of these trends is clear from your reading of this book. Your patients will surely benefit from your efforts, and you will benefit from a renewed sense of intellectual satisfaction and confidence throughout your career.